THE MAKING OF NURSE PROFESSIONALS

A TRANSFORMATIONAL, ETHICAL APPROACH

NANCY CRIGGER, PhD, MA, APRN, BC

Associate Professor
William Jewell College
Liberty, Missouri

NELDA GODFREY, PhD, ACNS-BC

Associate Dean for Undergraduate Programs
Clinical Associate Professor
School of Nursing
University of Kansas
Kansas City, Kansas

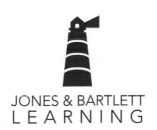

JONES & BARTLETT
LEARNING

World Headquarters
Jones & Bartlett Learning
40 Tall Pine Drive
Sudbury, MA 01776
978-443-5000
info@jblearning.com
www.jblearning.com

Jones & Bartlett Learning
Canada
6339 Ormindale Way
Mississauga, Ontario L5V 1J2
Canada

Jones & Bartlett Learning
International
Barb House, Barb Mews
London W6 7PA
United Kingdom

Jones & Bartlett Learning books and products are available through most bookstores and online booksellers. To contact Jones & Bartlett Learning directly, call 800-832-0034, fax 978-443-8000, or visit our website, www.jblearning.com.

Substantial discounts on bulk quantities of Jones & Bartlett Learning publications are available to corporations, professional associations, and other qualified organizations. For details and specific discount information, contact the special sales department at Jones & Bartlett Learning via the above contact information or send an email to specialsales@jblearning.com.

The authors, editor, and publisher have made every effort to provide accurate information. However, they are not responsible for errors, omissions, or for any outcomes related to the use of the contents of this book and take no responsibility for the use of the products and procedures described. Treatments and side effects described in this book may not be applicable to all people; likewise, some people may require a dose or experience a side effect that is not described herein. Drugs and medical devices are discussed that may have limited availability controlled by the Food and Drug Administration (FDA) for use only in a research study or clinical trial. Research, clinical practice, and government regulations often change the accepted standard in this field. When consideration is being given to use of any drug in the clinical setting, the health care provider or reader is responsible for determining FDA status of the drug, reading the package insert, and reviewing prescribing information for the most up-to-date recommendations on dose, precautions, and contraindications, and determining the appropriate usage for the product. This is especially important in the case of drugs that are new or seldom used.

Production Credits
Publisher: Kevin Sullivan
Acquisitions Editor: Amy Sibley
Associate Editor: Patricia Donnelly
Editorial Assistant: Rachel Shuster
Associate Production Editor: Katie Spiegel
Associate Marketing Manager: Katie Hennessy
V.P., Manufacturing and Inventory Control: Therese Connell

Composition: DataStream Content Solutions, LLC,
   Absolute Service Inc.
Cover Design: Scott Moden
Cover Image: © Robyn Mackenzie/ShutterStock, Inc.
Printing and Binding: Malloy, Inc.
Cover Printing: Malloy, Inc.

Library of Congress Cataloging-in-Publication Data
Crigger, Nancy.
   The making of nurse professionals: a transformational, ethical approach / Nancy Crigger, Nelda Godfrey.
      p. ; cm.
   Includes bibliographical references and index.
   ISBN 978-0-7637-8056-2 (pbk.)
   1. Nursing ethics. I. Godfrey, Nelda Schwinke, 1955- II. Title.
   [DNLM: 1. Ethics, Nursing. 2. Nurse's Role. WY 85 C928m 2011]
   RT85.C75 2011
   174.2—dc22
                                        2010017551
6048
Printed in the United States of America
14 13 12   10 9 8 7 6 5 4 3 2

Table of Contents

Foreword

Authors Nancy Crigger and Nelda Godfrey introduce a rich and thoughtful new book on ethics for nurses, nurse educators, and nurse administrators. It transcends the limited language of bioethics' principle-based ethics (Beauchamp & Childress, 2008) and addresses the problems with consumerist and bureaucratic approaches to educating nurses. They call for a transformational view of nurse education that changes from a narrow, technical, and professional approach to ethics to a view of formation for civic professionalism based upon the virtue tradition, the moral ideal of service to society, and human flourishing. The authors take a dialogical approach that will be controversial in some areas, but will enrich every reader's thinking on ethics in nursing practice. They also call for a change from transactional approaches to nursing education to a transformational approach. I consider both moves, the move from technical professionalism to civic professionalism and from transactional education to transformational education, essential to transforming nursing education.

Crigger and Godfrey embark on a bold venture to lay bare the limitations to ethics as it is taught in higher educational settings, pointing out that professional education, in general, and professional nursing education, in particular, demand more. The abandonment of a consumerist approach, which makes the student as an individual the center of nursing education, was done in favor of a more civic-based approach of calling for education to shape nursing education with the goal of developing good nurses for the sake of patients' human flourishing. In other words, they propose a practice-centered approach to nursing education rather than excessive focus on the student as a "consumer of education." In this sense, this book advocates a discipline-specific approach to nursing curricula and nursing pedagogies. The authors contend that the discipline is in the center, because the educator's chief responsibility is to the discipline in sufficiently preparing students to become *nurse professionals*, to become contributing members of the profession of nursing, and to serve society.

In Chapter 5 of this text, the authors introduce a promising new integrative, ethical Framework for Nurse Professionals (FrNP):

> ... the *moral agent* and the elements that the agent considers in determining how to live as a professional, *phronesis* or the process of deliberation, making fitting choices, and acting on those choices, and the *outcome*, or *telos* that impacts both the moral agent and the practice in which the agent is engaged. The FrNP represents the dynamic interplay of these elements as a life process that occurs over time. (p. 60)

In addition, they introduce the Stairstep Model of Professional Transformation:

> The FrNP is designed to communicate a unified model of deontology, consequentialism, and virtue ethics within a nursing context, showing movement and progress as the nurse grows as a nurse professional, all the while recognizing that no one is perfect and that the ideal cannot truly be achieved.... Three central ideas are communicated: (1) the place of principle-based ethics, consequentialist ethics and virtue ethics in professional

transformation; (2) the dynamic nature of flourishing and of making mistakes (slips); and (3) how a larger view of professional formation and transformation can help nursing students and nurses embrace a broader understanding of the discipline that is commensurate with the recognition and trust that nursing receives from society as a whole. (pp. 63–64)

Though I would argue that these frameworks might best be considered an integrated tool for drawing on multiple ethical frameworks, in some situations it is impossible to harmonize or integrate consequentialist and virtue ethics, and in turn it is highly doubtful that they should be considered hierarchical. These two models could be clarified and strengthened by adding clinical examples. Perhaps this will be done in a workbook or another future work. Nevertheless, their model is pluralistic and inclusive with a clear vision of the ends of good nursing practice.

In the Carnegie Study of Nursing Education (Benner, Sutphen, Leonard, & Day, 2010), students tell of the good they were trying to accomplish in their rich narratives of pivotal learning in practice: meeting the patient as a person; preserving dignity and personhood of patient; responding to substandard practice; advocating for patients; and engaging fully in learning to do "good" nursing practice. These notions of good nursing practice organized the concerns of nursing student narratives of their pivotal learning in clinical practice during their education. Students in the National Carnegie Nursing Education Study also used *calling, notions of good*, and the centrality of a *self-improving practice* to describe their clinical nursing education in particular:

> In both interviews and survey responses, advanced-level students and beginning nurses frequently described the way in which their sense of mission, or *calling*, made it possible for them to withstand the rigors of learning for practice and gave them the courage to enter high-stakes situations, where the consequence of a mistake can be enormous. The students claim that this understanding of the significance of their work and their identification with nursing practice were what kept them focused through terrifying clinical situations, heavy or conflicting academic demands, or competing family and work responsibilities—any of which might have led them to drop out. They cite classmates who were performing well but who did not identify themselves with the significance and relevance of [good] nursing practice and consequently chose to drop out of the program. (Benner et al., 2010, p. 178)

Crigger and Godfrey declare that, "No discipline can be rich if its members are marooned in a stagnated or underdeveloped point of view. The academic discipline and profession of nursing can only benefit from a wider view. Colleagues in arts and sciences and in other disciplines can broaden our own understanding of the nursing profession." I applaud their broader view of ethics and greater emphasis on the role of the humanities and the virtue tradition (Benner et al., 2010) in the formation of student nurses. As Dunne (1997) observes, "A practice is not just a surface on which one can display instant virtuosity. It grounds one in a tradition that has been formed through an elaborate development and that exists at any juncture only in the dispositions (slowly and perhaps painfully acquired) of its recognized practitioners" (p. 378).

In sum, I enthusiastically recommend this book for student nurses, for nurses in general, as well as for nurse educators, administrators, and leaders. It will go a long way toward a badly needed enrichment and invigoration of nursing ethics, nursing curricula, and pedagogies. This book is highly recommended for all those nursing courses called: "Issues in Nursing," "Nursing Ethics," "Advanced Nursing Practice," and nursing policy courses linked to ethical discourse. The book is a significant new contribution to nursing education, administration, and practice.

Patricia Benner, PhD, RN, FAAN
Professor Emerita
University of California, San Francisco School of Nursing
Department of Social and Behavioral Sciences
San Francisco, California

Senior Scholar for The Carnegie Foundation
for the Advancement of Teaching
Stanford, California

REFERENCES

Beauchamp, T. L., & Childress, J. F. (2008) *Principles of bioethics*. New York: Oxford University Press.

Benner, P., Sutphen, M., Leonard, V., & Day, L. (2010) *Educating nurses: A call for radical transformation*. San Francisco: Jossey-Bass and Stanford, CA: The Carnegie Foundation for the Advancement of Teaching.

Dunne, J. (1997). *Back to the rough ground: Practical judgement and the lure of technique*. Notre Dame, IN: University of Notre Dame Press.

Introduction

"Students," one seasoned nurse bemoaned, "just aren't what they used to be. It isn't like when *we were students.*" Our outspoken nurse was correct on a number of levels; nursing education was different, students were different, and practice was different. Nurses were struggling to birth a profession and now struggle to birth professionals of good moral character who can fit societal need. The world has moved from the nostalgia of an age gone by to contemporary nursing practice of today that Benner, Sutphen, Leonard, and Day (2010) claim is under "enormous pressure of expanded expectations" (p. 1).

Professional education has become increasingly difficult in the contemporary nursing world. Curricular emphasis on knowledge development, a narrow interpretation of ethics, and the socially constructed professional have eclipsed character development and the transformational nature of professional development. Nursing students often graduate with knowledge of drug interactions, patient safety, and symptom management but with only a vague sense of how to be a professional and how to view professional growth as an essential part of their career.

Like many other professions, expert practitioners, educators, and theorists, nurse leaders increasingly recognize that the current system is insufficient to do the work required for a professional education (Doane, Pauly, Brown, & McPherson, 2004; Vezeau, 2006). The authors, who are also part of this awakening, are firmly convinced that a richer and more robust understanding of professionalism than is currently taught will substantially improve nursing education. Any curriculum, we determined, must be comprehensive, flexible enough to respond to change, but firm enough in its philosophical and conceptual foundations to support the fundamental changes that are necessary for student nurses to become true professionals.

In the quest for a richer conception of professionalism, the authors reconsidered professionalism, professional ethics, and ethics. Professionalism is more than just the contemporary social conception of nurses as professionals whose sole value is measured through meeting role expectations and following rules. Professional nurses, if only understood from a social perspective, become empty uniforms whose value is placed in what they do rather than who they are. Nurses are individuals with character and substance, who live real lives as professionals. Therefore, it is crucial that nursing education address individual character development as fundamental for meeting both personal and social expectations of the professional nurse. Character development as a substantive part of professional education has remained part of the hidden curriculum and had been all but abandoned by most disciplines as a explicit part of professional curricula. Fortunately, because the problem of the "empty uniform" is being further exposed, character development is reemerging as a priority. These changes have also opened a broader view of professional ethics. Virtue ethics that stress character development have been revived—and taken center stage.

After a philosophical inquiry into the nature and scope of professionalism and extensive review of current literature from many disciplines, the authors developed a comprehensive framework and a dynamic model of professional development that we hope will fill the gap. The Framework for Nurse Professionals (FrNP) synthesizes many elements from different sources: moral psychology, ethical traditions, professional ethics, and professional theory. The Stairstep Model of Professional Transformation underscores the dynamic nature of professionalism as a lifelong process.

The book content poses and ultimately answers these three questions:

What is the nature of a profession and of nurse professionals?
Is it possible to develop an inclusive ethical framework for nurse professionals?
How can professionalism be taught?

A few definitions will help readers avoid the quicksand of language ambiguity. Some ethicists make distinctions between moral and ethical. However, no such distinction is made in this book; ethical and moral are used synonymously. As nurse ethicists, the authors distinguish between nurse professional and professional nurse. By nurse professional we mean a person who professes to be a member of the discipline and has individual qualities or characteristics that inform and motivate him or her to make good moral choices. A nurse professional becomes a professional nurse through validation by examination or by institutional verification.

The profession is a collective body of persons who profess to practice a calling or vocation that is recognized by certain sociopolitical and legal bodies to enjoy special privileges that includes some degree of autonomy, but from whom special obligations are required (Crigger, 2009; Morin & Green, 2007). Professionalism is understood as the qualities of an individual that enable an individual to be distinguished as a professional and, in nursing, a nurse professional.

The contents of the book are unique to the literature in nursing and are expected to be controversial. We welcome, and in fact relish, controversial response. Progress in nursing and in nursing education is not made by a watershed phenomenon in which everyone agrees but, rather, by dissent, by a chipping away, by a winnowing, to determine what best fits and what does not. As the authors, we believe that the reader will find at least some modicum of fresh, bold thought to be chipped away at in this book.

Although discussion in the book is strongly influenced by our Western heritage, the discussion promotes deeper thinking about nursing as a discipline and its relationship to recipients of care, to local society, and to the wider global society. We hope that this project contributes to the making of a nurse professional through education and through a lifelong process of transformation. As nurse educators we hope to contribute some small piece to the *making* of *nurse professionals* now and in generations to come.

REFERENCES

Benner, P., Sutphen, M., Leonard, V., & Day, L. (2010). *Educating nurses: A call for radical transformation.* San Francisco: Jossey-Bass and Stanford, CA: The Carnegie Foundation for the Advancement of Teaching.

Crigger, N. J. (2009). Toward understanding the nature of conflict of interest and application to the discipline of nursing. *Nursing Philosophy, 10,* 253–262.

Doane, G., Pauly, B., Brown, H., & McPherson, G. (2004). Exploring the heart of ethical nursing practice. *Nursing Ethics, 11*(3), 240–251.

Morin, K., & Green, S. K. (2007). Professionalism in biomedical science. *American Journal of Bioethics, 7*(2), 66–68.

Vezeau, T. M. (2006). Teaching professional values in a BSN program. *International Journal of Nursing Scholarship, 3*(1), 1–15.

Acknowledgments

Achievements are rarely accomplished in isolation. Both of us, as authors and more importantly as people, are grateful for the benefits we have received from others.

Nancy was given an opportunity—through failure—to accomplish a second master's degree in philosophy at the University of Florida. Dr. R. M. Hare profoundly influenced her to understand philosophy and to see excellence in professionalism incarnate. Nancy's brother, Dr. James Jones, a physician and ethicist, has provided lifelong encouragement, support, and wisdom.

Nelda worked closely with exemplary direct care nurses during 21 years of prn bedside practice in inner-city hospitals. These colleagues provided tremendous insights on *what it means to be a nurse professional*. Special thanks to her academic mentors, Susan Taylor and Kit Smith, her nursing and liberal studies colleagues at William Jewel College, particularly Dale Kuehne and Gary Armstrong, the University of Kansas School of Nursing for its support and resources, and the University of Kansas Hospital Professionalism Council for its willingness to serve as a crucible in envisioning the best in professional nursing practice. Sincere thanks as well to the Liberty Hospital Ethics Committee and the University of Kansas Hospital Ethics Committee, the Center for Practical Bioethics, and especially to Dr. Robert Lyman Potter, senior research associate at the time, whose mentoring often made the difference in taking that next step forward.

Our gratitude to those people who helped move inchoate ideas to a finished product: Dr. Lygia Holcomb, David Martin, Mary Meyer, Michelle Septer, Sally Barhydt, and Deb Navedo all of whom provided careful and thoughtful review of the manuscript. The editorial staff from Jones & Bartlett Learning was excellent in transforming the early drafts into publishable form. Finally, we owe a great deal to the authors from all disciplines from whom we learned.

SECTION 1

What Is the Nature of a Profession and of Nurse Professionals?

CHAPTER 1

Professionalism in Nursing: An Overview

If we set about bringing up our child . . . we shall have to bring him up
to have not merely a policy or practice of obeying these principles but firm
dispositions of character which accord with them.

—R. M. HARE, 1989

The increasing incidence of unethical and illegal scandals in recent years and the growing erosion of public trust in professionals has led experts in the field to agree that there is a "crisis of professionalism" (Sullivan, 2005). Leaders in many professions believe that the proliferation of scandals and poor professional image are a result of failure within the professional educational systems to educate professionals properly (Coulehan, Williams, McCreary, & Belling, 2003).

As educators and ethicists, our purpose in writing this book is to strengthen professional nursing education by reframing professionalism and professional ethics as parts of a transformational process of individual development that, when combined with other ethical traditions, forms a framework to better educate students to become nurse professionals. This first chapter sets the stage for subsequent chapters by presenting a brief overview of ethical traditions, assumptions that are foundational to the framework presented in Chapter 5, and a brief synopsis of each chapter.

PROBLEMS OF PROFESSIONAL EDUCATION

In recent years, and especially in disciplines that are regulated by examination, curricula are heavy in content related to competency education with little time allotted for more subjects that are less critical or "fluffy," like professional ethics or professionalism. What *is* taught may be either part of the hidden or implicit curriculum or marginalized by merging professionalism and professional ethics in other subject areas like bioethics, management, or leadership (Day, 2005; Harris, 2008; Sullivan, 2005).

Professionalism is often limited to meeting social expectations by following rules, policies, and codes. The sociological paradigm of professionalism has emerged as dominant and almost exclusive in contemporary society as what Barker (1992) called the complex sociological definition. According to Barker, most experts on the subject of professionalism define professionals—legally, economically, and socially—as a *group* of individuals who have certain obligations to society. The professional agent as an individual with character and virtues was, in recent decades, marginalized or excluded altogether.

The sociological paradigm has not always held supreme status in nursing education and professional nursing organizations in the United States. Earlier education and writings in nursing stressed the importance of development of character and good qualities in the individual nurse. Nightingale, for example, spoke of character development of the nurse, the nurse's commitment to seek personal moral excellence and to live a life of purity.

However, as the sociological paradigm became more dominant, the perception of the nurse as an individual with morally relevant psychological traits diminished as a topic of discussion in education but remained alive as word remnants. Words like character, moral qualities, moral excellence, ideal self, or virtue persisted in our language of ethics and professionalism to remind us that there is something more to professionalism in nursing than social expectations. With no clear commitment to a psychological paradigm and character development, the nurse professional became an empty uniform with nobody inside, a doer of work who fulfilled a social role rather than a person of moral agency, integrity, and excellence.

Healthcare ethics, like professionalism and professional ethics, has also been dominated by the social paradigm that focuses on decision-making processes justified through a deontology or consequentialism tradition. Dissatisfaction with the current state of healthcare ethics has led experts from many disciplines, including nursing, to express concern and to consider alternatives.

Two alternatives to the current established healthcare ethic in nursing have been suggested. The first is to assume that ethics in nursing is so unique in nature that it requires a purely nursing theory to address professionalism and nursing practice. This unique strategy has paralleled feminist theory and advocates two elements that are not part of other ethical theory traditions: the ontological basis of the human condition is relational and partiality of nursing care is acceptable. Partiality of treatment, treatment because one cares rather than because of fairness, is particularly troublesome. An exclusive ethic of care and its impact on professional ethics denies the value of traditional moral theories to participate in moral discourse and has been shown by many to be philosophically and conceptually insufficient as a stand-alone moral theory (Crigger, 1997; Kuhse, 1993; Veatch, 1998).

A second suggested strategy for improving healthcare ethics is to be inclusive: preserve the richness of ethical theory traditions but add virtue ethics and include other, more contemporary, elements (Begley, 2005; McCarthy, 2006). We, the authors, advocate the second strategy of preserving ethical traditions as a more realistic and fruitful way of approaching ethics and professional ethics in nursing in particular. The need for a richer conceptualization of professionalism parallels the need for a more comprehensive and inclusive healthcare ethic for nursing.

ETHICAL THEORY TRADITIONS

The three main traditions of moral theory are consequentialism, deontological or principled ethics, and virtue ethics. With marginalization of virtue ethics and individual moral character development, the language and substance of morality has become fragmented and the essence of it, according to MacIntyre (1981), lost.

MacIntyre (1981) also saw fragmentation as a result of the historical shaping of traditions. Centuries of moral discourse accompanied these traditions and each tradition has been subjected to modification from advocates and critics alike. Recipients of these traditions can only acknowledge that there are limitations to understanding the traditions and that they, in turn, add their own perceptions. Table 1-1 and Figure 1-1 offer further, simplified comparisons of the three ethical traditions.

Table 1-1   A Comparison of Virtue, Consequentialism, and Deontological Ethical Traditions

Tradition	Virtue	Consequentialism	Deontology
Ethical question	How shall we live?	How shall we decide?	How shall we decide?
Justification of ethic	Personal/psychological Good and the good of all equates with ethical	Decisions for the best outcomes for all equates with ethical	Decisions for the agent to do duty and base it on sound principles; motive equates with ethical
Justice	Exercises judgment in particular cases, phronesis Claim what is due; Christian impartiality and golden rule	Each one counts as one and receives equal burden and benefit	Categorical imperative; universalizability during 20th century[†]
Paradigm approximated	Psychological	Sociological	Sociological
Ethic defined	Method to enable human beings to understand and transform their essential nature*	Method of making better or right moral decisions	Method of making right moral decisions
Problematic issues identified	Virtues and other elements of tradition are loosely conceptualized Less clear sense of justice	Less room for individual justice	Not contextualized and less related to outcomes

*MacIntyre (1981).
†Hare (1989).

Figure 1-1   Scope of ethical traditions.

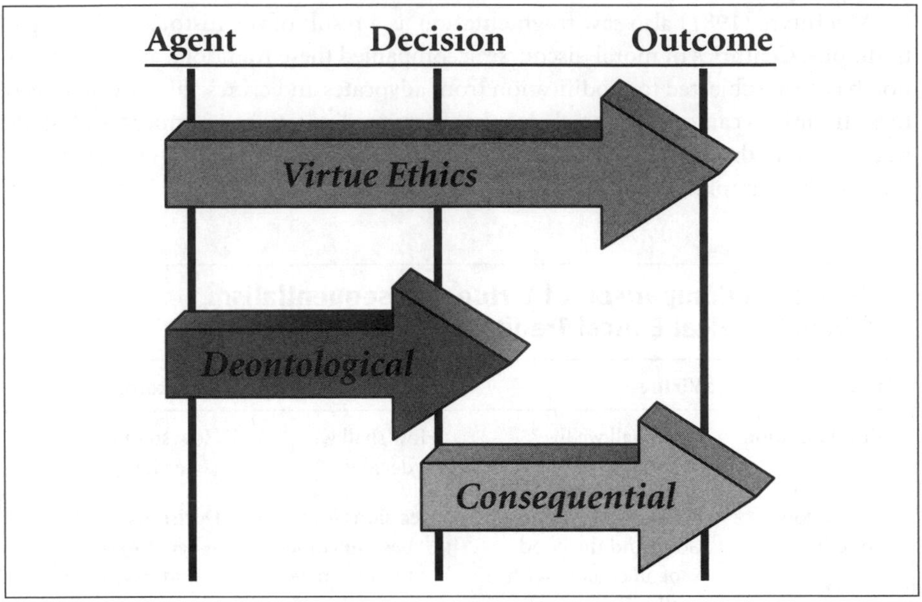

The limited scope of ethics and professionalism relates, in part, to the presentation of these traditions as starkly differing ethical world views. A more complete interpretation of the ethical traditions is that they are complex systems of thought that are both distinct and similar to other traditions. For example, justice is an ethical thread that is common to ethical traditions. The golden rule, Kant's categorical imperative, each counts as one rule in utilitarianism, or the more contemporary view of justice as critical thinking in a process called universalizability (Hare, 1989) are all ways of viewing justice but from differing traditions. Recognizing the similarities in theory traditions and adding the missing pieces would enrich ethics, professional ethics, and healthcare ethics.

Consequentialism

Consequentialism describes a group of theories that use the outcome of a decision as the measure of ethical appropriateness. Utilitarian theory, the best known of the consequentialist theories, is based on one principle: The goal of human activity should impartially promote the welfare and interests of others so that the greatest happiness or pleasure is achieved for the greatest number. Consequentialist theories justify decisions through the outcome. There is no refutation of the outcomes as morally relevant in ethical choice. A number of weaknesses can be identified if consequentialism is used solely as the determinant in moral decisions. The chief problem with consequentialism is that there are no limits to the methods that can be used to obtain outcomes as long as the outcomes are beneficial. Some shady practices might produce good outcomes if taken to the extreme. Lying, stealing, and even murder can be morally acceptable if the consequences are beneficial enough.

Deontology

Deontological ethical theories, also called duty bound or principled ethical theories, have exerted a strong influence on healthcare ethics in the United States. A principled ethic justifies decisions made based on conforming to one's duty to act on universal laws, principles, or rules. Kantian ethics includes the idea of impartiality or universalizability that is evident in the different expressions of the categorical imperative. Deontology has been criticized because this tradition is contextually disconnected and because there is inherent weakness for solving dilemmas or conflict between or among principles. Ethical appropriateness is based on following rules, respecting rights, doing one's duty—not on outcomes. Taken in its purist sense, the deontological tradition disconnects the decision maker from the real world. Obligations or duties stated as principles are also notorious for an inability to facilitate decisions. If a person has two or more duties, then a decision must be made about which one of the duties or principles should take precedence.

For example, Nurse P has an appointment to meet with her colleague at a specified time. She has a duty to show up and keep her promise. On the way to the meeting, she stops to assist an automobile crash victim because she has a duty to be beneficent to others but, in doing so, Nurse P misses the meeting. Nurse P, using deontological ethics, is forced to decide which of the duties should take precedence.

Virtue Ethics

Virtue ethics, the third type of moral tradition, is central to our view of professionalism and the Framework for Nurse Professionals (FrNP) and is presented in Chapter 5. Aristotle was the early proponent of virtue ethics. The natural desire of any species—human or animal—according to Aristotle is to produce a state of doing and being well. Virtues are qualities or characteristics that are developed by individuals that, when acted on in a balanced way, are morally praiseworthy and *reinforce acting in the same way in the future*. The function of virtues is conceptualized through Aristotle's doctrine of the mean: Virtues are a continuum for which the right action is the prudent or temperate choice between two extremes and one that is fitting to the situation (Aristotle, trans 1998, Chase translation).

Aristotle believed that wisdom and prudence were, in themselves, virtues that helped an agent make good ethical decisions. For example, generosity is often identified as a virtue. One can be too generous or give too much whereas, on the other hand, one can be stingy. Being generous is, according to Aristotle, using the virtue well and that is ". . . to feel them at the right times, with reference to the right objects, towards the right people with the right motive, and in the right way . . ." (Aristotle, trans 1998, Chase translation 1106b, 14–24). This sustained and repeated proper exercise of one's choices builds character in the individual and reinforces the individual to himself or herself and to others as a virtuous person.

MacIntyre's classic work, *After Virtue* (1981), brought a new awareness of the fragmented state of contemporary ethics and made a clear argument for the inclusion of virtue ethics in moral discourse. Virtue ethics is continuing to gain popularity in many disciplines because it addresses the individual agent and the agent's ability to participate in a transformational process (Begley, 2005; Pellegrino & Thomasma, 1993). However, virtue ethics, like consequentialism and deontology, is not without criticism. What is "good" is obscure and the problem of deciding what is good falls to the imprecise measuring stick of the doctrine of the mean. Second, virtues themselves create problems, because by their nature they are elusive and only indirectly empirically measurable. Virtues are clearly not universal in many cases and depend on culture, gender, historical periods, generational groups, and to the professions individually.

INTEGRATION OF ETHICAL TRADITIONS

Of the three ethical theory traditions, virtue ethics, is most central to our framework because it is comprehensive and it emphasizes development of the individual. Deontological ethical traditions are consistent with the social paradigm whereas consequentialist theory tradition is characterized by justification through outcomes.

According to Pellegrino (2005), there are three approaches to virtue ethics: the thick version that claims that all ethics are virtue based, the thin version that makes virtue ethics only one among many theories of ethics with no edge to any other, and the complementary version. The virtue ethic tradition proposed through the FrNP falls somewhere in between thick and thin. We advocate for an inclusive ethic but set the virtue ethic tradition as the primary ethic of professionalism. Because professionalism so closely relates to ethics, the framework for educating nurse professionals has a double effect. A framework structures thought, evidence, theory, and values so that one understands and acts on this understanding (Barnes, 2002). The FrNP provides the conceptual basis for professionalism but is inclusive of the three ethic traditions.

ASSUMPTIONS

Ontology of the Framework

There are assumptions about the individual and about psychological responses that are key to understanding the framework. *The fundamental ontological element is the existence of individual qua individual who has the ability to choose to act in a certain way.*

Freedom to make choices is fundamental to ethical endeavors. Without choice, all decisions are determined and therefore there is no alternative and no ability to be ethical. To illustrate, Nurse L is attacked and robbed upon leaving work. This crime may be a wanton act or perhaps she was targeted by someone who knew her. In either case, the perpetrator had a choice of whether or not to commit the crime. The crime is a moral and a legal breach of what is expected from a member of a society. Nurse L had a choice about walking at that particular place at that particular time. Let us say that most people aware of personal safety would be prudent enough to avoid this situation. In fact, she was breaking the rules of the hospital by not asking for security to accompany her to her car. Nurse L, we might claim, did not use prudence in choosing to walk at that time and place and neglected hospital policy. Nurse L's decision and action, in this context, may have moral significance.

Goal of Professional Nursing

Nurse professionals make choices with the goal of being a good nurse professional and doing good work. Good choices are choices that are ethically defensible and that benefit the individual making them, people for whom service is provided, and/or the common good of society. As professionals our choices promote patient and societal interests above our own self-interests (Crigger, 2009). Corporately, if individuals of good character come together to form social bonds, the social institutions will result in political and social establishments that promote the good of all.

In nursing, the ability to come together and socially determine the aggregate good for our discipline's members is closely linked to what has been called the metaparadigm domains of nurse, health, patient, and environment (Parker & Smith, 2010). This broad conceptualization of structure allows room for change in the contents of the terminology. The discipline has distinguished itself by promoting a more comprehensive view of health that includes disease but is not limited to it. More recently, the enhancement therapies that modify physical traits (e.g., plastic surgery or chemical treatment) or enhance performance (e.g., the medications that increase physical sexual response or drugs that increase growth of children) have moved into the scope of care. Are enhancement therapies promoting health?

Perhaps in the future, the discipline will address more clearly and distinctly the novel issues that challenge our definitions of health or how enhancement and technology impact social justice and especially global social justice.

The Nature of Character

Character is part of an individual's psychological self that is developed through a lifelong process to the extent to which the individual is capable. The pervasive view that moral development and character are only established in early childhood has not been supported by research. Adulthood, especially young adulthood, is an active and engaging time for establishing marriage or intimate long-term relationships, parenting, and successfully negotiating a new professional role. During these transitional times of adulthood, development of character may be particularly influenced (Piper, Gentile, & Parks, 1993). The more contemporary, dynamic view of moral and character development is also a presupposition that individuals can learn and change from experiences of wrongdoing (Martin, 1999).

Good Character Can Be Developed

Formation of a good character or the ability to act virtuously results from, at least initially, personal discipline and guidance from outside the individual. If good character is the result of developing the virtues or abilities to make good choices, as Aristotle claimed, then ethics can be taught. Medical students, according to Leach (2004), enter their professional education with a high degree of altruism but lack professionalism. The professional is one who becomes able, during the educational process, to be "habitually faithful to professional values in highly complex situations" (Leach, 2004, p. 12). This assumption does not refer to an educational system that controls access to knowledge or indoctrinates students, but rather refers to the ability of an individual to develop right attitudes, to be guided to make choices that are good, and to act in such a way that is consistent with the moral codes and standards of the discipline.

Professional Ideals

The goal of professionalism in nursing is to enable nurses to flourish through participation in a transformational process that aspires toward professional ideals and that seeks the highest good for care recipients, community, and themselves. Traditional ethics, as MacIntyre (1981) claimed, has been viewed narrowly as disagreements between and among ethical points of view when making decisions. Ethical tradition addresses much more than just the immediacy and shortsightedness of decision making. If traditions of ethics or any quasi-ethical nursing theory are working, they are working well if they function as a guide and a moral compass that offers (1) validation when a choice is morally praiseworthy or (2) caution when it is not.

Ethics, when distilled into determining a solution to a moral dilemma, misses the most significant work of ethical thinking. Singer (1993) expressed the primary question of ethics, the broader overarching question of ethics, in the title of his book, *How Are We to Live?* Yes, we use ethical thinking in daily decisions, but if we only consider ethics as a means for making decisions we are shortsighted and miss the bigger picture and the richness of ethics as a dynamic way of living our daily lives.

Ethics as a Transition to the Good

Ethics is the method by which human beings understand how to transform from a natural state into individuals who seek the highest good. Contemporary ethics has been most closely associated with ethical decision making that is justified by context and/or by ethical theories. There is a wide range of how people use the term *ethic*. For example, Hare (1989) defined ethics as a branch of logic and the study of moral argument to discern how to answer questions rationally. Grace (2009) defined ethics as simply "philosophical inquiry about the good" (p. 409). MacIntyre's (1981) conceptualized ethics, which is inclusive of virtue ethical thought, is more comprehensive than either of the two; for MacIntyre, ethics is the power of thought and practice that transforms human beings to move beyond the human state to be and do good.

ORGANIZATION AND FOCUS OF THE BOOK

To address professional education in nursing, this book is organized around three essential questions in need of thoughtful answers.

What is the nature of a profession and of nurse professionals?
Is it possible to develop an inclusive ethical framework for nurse professionals?
How can professionalism be taught?

The first question is addressed in Chapters 2 and 3. Chapter 2 is an in-depth exploration of the current status of professionalism in nursing. The authors closely look at what is traditionally meant by a profession and its historical traditions. The etymology of the word is explicated, and it is argued that no word is synonymous with professionalism in all senses—the word *professional* has a unique meaning. The final section explores the two paradigms of professionalism and our philosophical position about professionalism is explained.

The impoverished state of professional education that has been identified in a number of disciplines unfolds in Chapter 3. There are social and political forces that have historically influenced and prohibited the robust teaching of professionalism.

The response to the second question is explicated by first addressing professionalism and its historical roots in nursing, and by a more in-depth discussion of the fundamental aspects of virtue ethics tradition. The content in Chapter 4 is a description of the historical development of virtue ethics; professionalism in nursing is presented along with a synopsis of the more contemporary virtue theory. Chapter 5 introduces the fundamental elements of the FrNP and the Stairstep Model of Professional Transformation. Further discussion of the benefits of using a more comprehensive and clearly explicated framework is also presented.

Our final question, how can professionalism be taught?, is answered in the remaining chapters. Chapter 6 is an account of the recent activity and new initiatives that have been launched by other disciplines, such as medicine and law, to improve professional education. General and specific ways to approach curriculum development as well as specific strategies for course structure, instruction methods, and individual education that are most compatible with the FrNP and virtue ethics are presented.

In Chapter 7, we turn to ways of evaluating professional development in the education program and beyond. There are a number of crucial questions that emerge. Are educators able to measure students' progress in developing moral character and professionalism? Can criteria be used to select better candidates for admission that are not based solely on scholarship, but rather on the student's proclivity and openness to moral education or to evaluating an existing moral character? Does the cognitive dissonance experienced between the educational program and students' clinical perceptions of nurse professionals impact student development of moral excellence (Coulehan, et al., 2003)? And finally, how or what methodology is most fitting for use with the FrNP framework?

Virtues that are significant but perhaps more often relegated to the hidden curriculum are given a closer look in relation to the discipline of nursing in Chapter 8. The chapter discussion begins with a more in-depth review of virtues that is followed by the presentation of four virtues that are believed to be central to nursing professionals. Compassion and integrity are well-known, while bravery and humility are rarely addressed yet are fundamental to the profession.

The final chapter, Chapter 9, is a presentation of the possible elements that will impact the trajectory of professional education. No futurist musing would be complete without considering the challenges faced by our profession and recognizing that education is shaped by future needs of society. There is a wealth of issues currently emerging for future contemplation and a wide variation in global views of professionalism. We have only begun to consider the future impact from and on transcultural and transglobal nursing (Davis, Tschudin, & de Raeve, 2006; Hirschfeld, 2006). Although a thorough discussion of professionalism and what professional means to nurses from other cultures is beyond our scope, a number of studies related to nurse professionalism are already part of the international nursing literature. To illustrate, the extension of distance learning has had an incredible impact on the education of nurse professionals. Does socialization online work effectively to develop moral excellence and professionalism? And, finally, the role of nurses is expanding globally. Advanced practice is not particular to the United States but a global phenomenon (Sheer & Wong, 2008). What issues will emerge from the reshaping of nurses' authority and responsibility?

REFERENCES

Barker, S. F. (1992). What is a profession? *Professional Ethics, 1*(1–2), 73–99.

Barnes, L. (2002). Reflective Christian communication in moral controversies. *Business & Professional Ethics Journal, 21*(3–4), 151–170.

Begley, A. M. (2005). Practicing virtue: A challenge to the view that a virtue centered approach to ethics lacks practical content. *Nursing Ethics, 12*(6), 622–637.

Coulehan, J., Williams, P. C., McCreary, V., & Belling, C. (2003). The best lack all conviction: Biomedical ethics, professionalism, and social responsibilities. *Cambridge Quarterly of Healthcare Ethics, 12*, 21–38.

Crigger, N. J. (1997). Why caring doesn't work: A review of eight arguments against an ethic of care. *Journal of Professional Nursing, 13*(4), 217–221.

Crigger, N. J. (2009). Toward understanding the nature of conflict of interest and application to the discipline of nursing. *Nursing Philosophy, 10*, 253–262.

Davis, A. J., Tschudin, V., & de Raeve, L. (2006). The future: Teaching nursing ethics. In A. J. Davis, V. Tschudin, & L. Tew (Eds.), *Essentials of teaching and learning nursing ethics* (pp. 339–352). London: Churchill Livingston.

Day, L. (2005). Nursing practice and civic professionalism. *American Journal of Critical Care, 14*, 434–437.

Grace, P. J. (2009). *Nursing ethics and professional responsibility in advanced practice.* Sudbury, MA: Jones and Bartlett.

Hare, R. M. (1989). *Moral thinking.* Oxford, UK: Clarendon Press.

Harris, C. E. (2008). The good engineer: Giving virtue its due in engineering ethics. *Science Engineering Ethics, 14*(2), 153–164.

Hirschfeld, M. (2006). An international perspective. In A. J. Davis, V. Tschudin, & L. Tew (Eds.), *Essentials of teaching and learning nursing ethics.* London: Churchill Livingston.

Kuhse, H. (1993). Caring is not enough: Reflections on a nursing ethics of care. *The Australian Journal of Advanced Nursing, 11*(1), 32–42.

Leach, D. C. (2004). Professionalism: The formation of physicians. *American Journal of Bioethics, 4*(2), 11–12.

MacIntyre, A. (1981). *After virtue: A study in moral theory.* Notre Dame, IN: University of Notre Dame Press.

Martin, M. (1999). Explaining wrongdoing in professions. *Journal of Social Philosophy, 30*(2), 232–250.

McCarthy, J. (2006). A pluralist view of nursing ethics. *Nursing Philosophy, 7*, 157–164.

Parker, M. E., & Smith, M. C. (2010). *Nursing theories and nursing practice* (3rd ed.). Philadelphia: F. A. Davis Company.

Pellegrino, E. D. (2005). Professionalism, profession and the virtues of the good physician. *The Mount Sinai Journal of Medicine, 69*(6), 378–384.

Pellegrino, E. D., & Thomasma, D. C. (1993). *The virtues in medical practice.* New York: Oxford University Press.

Piper, T. R., Gentile, M. C., & Parks, S. D. (1993). *Can ethics be taught?* Boston: Harvard Business School.

Sheer, B., & Wong, F. K. (2008). The development of advanced nursing practice globally. *Journal of Nursing Scholarship, 40*(3), 204–211.

Singer, P. (1993). *How are we to live?* Melbourne, Australia: The Text Publishing Company.

Sullivan, W. M. (2005). *Work and integrity* (2nd ed.). San Francisco: Jossey-Bass.

Veatch, R. M. (1998). The place of care in ethical theory. *Journal of Medicine and Philosophy, 23*(2), 210–224.

CHAPTER 2

The Crises in Professionalism and Professional Education

*. . . the language and the appearances of morality persist even though
the integral substance of morality has to a large degree been fragmented
and then in part destroyed.*

—ALASDAIR MACINTYRE, 1981

The trend in contemporary society in the United States, according to Sullivan (2005), is a growing mistrust of the professions. Public trust in many professions is diminishing and there is every indication that this decline may be justified. Public mistrust has been fueled by widespread wrongdoing that fall into two main categories. Either professionals place self-serving interests before their commitment to serve others or professionals take advantage of their privileged status (Coulehan, Williams, McCreary, & Belling, 2003).

But what, besides obvious wrongful acts, accounts for the ailing view of professionalism? The contemporary view of professionalism has been shaped by many diverse forces. The semantic and social factors that contribute to the current difficulties in professionalism appear in the first section of this chapter. The following section is a description of the two professional paradigms that undergird contemporary perceptions of professionalism. The final sections examine the current state of the more evident contributing factors to the professional education and suggest a more inclusive approach to professionalism and professional ethics.

STATUS OF CONTEMPORARY PROFESSIONALISM

There appears to be no end to media reports of fraud, personal indiscretions, conflicts of interest, tax evaders promoted to high public office, and voter fraud. Some professionals and professions who hold power through public influence, like journalists, have also come under scrutiny. Journalists are ethically responsible to report information objectively but that obligation may be compromised by political and personal views (Luebke, 1989). Public distrust of the mainstream media has resulted, at least in part, in the development and success of alternative media sources that claim to present more objective reporting in the United States.

Other sources of misconduct occur because of monetary gain. The shift of the business model into all public sectors and into health care also takes some responsibility for professional image decline. In earlier decades, the traditional service/fiduciary model was the dominant social model. But, in recent years, the business model with the lure of profit may at times overpower even the most ethical people and agencies. The public's view of professionals has also changed to one that is consumer centered. An entitlement mentality of business has created unrealistic public expectations of a professional's responsibility (Bottery, 1995; Conrad, 2007). No discipline, no one professional, and no institution has been immune from ultimate public scrutiny and the disenchantment that occurs through the many reports of professional failings.

From the historical perspective, a fragmentation of professional and personal roles, a more self-oriented society, and the decline of cohesion within professional groups have influenced professionals. These changes have likewise influenced the public. The exposure of errors in health care has eroded the public's trust (Crigger, 2005). Professionals in some disciplines have been particularly hard-hit and have lost the trust and favor of society, whereas other disciplines like nursing and firefighters may have gained public favor (Chadwick & Thompson, 2000; Davis, 2001; Yam, 2004). Even though nursing as a profession has a favorable public image, there is no indication that this public favor will be sustainable in light of the changes in health care and in nursing that are currently in progress.

In nursing, advanced practice roles are shaping and being shaped by societal needs (Ford, 2008; Klein, 2008). Nursing education has had dramatic changes in student access and in the variety of program opportunities in higher education. The entire US healthcare system may undergo dramatic changes over the next few years and decades. Electronic medical records, healthcare reform, government financial insolvency, and advancing technology are only a few of the many forces that will promote change. And, more recently, the worldwide economic slump may bring future changes that, in the past, have not been even imagined.

In view of the troubled professions and tremendous societal changes, it may be a proper time for nursing, as a profession, to follow the lead of many other professions in reevaluating the profession and professionalism. What are the fundamental elements of the profession and how should each nurse act as a professional? Has the traditional model of nursing professionalism been reshaped already and have we have lost something of value from earlier conceptions of professionalisms? Or, on the other extreme, does our profession embrace a model of professionalism that is outmoded and inappropriate for today's world?

THE SEMANTICS OF PROFESSIONALISM IN NURSING

Although the discipline has historically struggled to be accepted by society and by other professions as a profession, confusion remains over the actual meaning of professional in nursing (Liaschenko & Peter, 2004). If we were to ask a nurse for a definition of *professional*, perhaps the issue will be clearer. Nurse H works 12-hour shifts in a busy general surgical unit. He graciously agrees to spend a minute conversing. When we ask, "What is a nurse professional?," he first responds with a puzzled look. He asks for clarification and then gives a vague response. "It means that nurses have a defined scope of practice and that they are licensed by the state to work." This limited response is no surprise; what is most significant is least explicit. The word *professional* has deep meaning for nurses' identities and is central to the discipline, but remains elusive to sufficient articulation.

In fact *professional* and *profession* often appear in some of our discipline's most significant documents. The American Association of Colleges of Nursing's (AACN; 2008) *The Essentials of Baccalaureate Education for Professional Nursing Practice* identifies *professionalism and professional values* as one of eight essentials in the newly revised guidelines. Each word in the word cloud (Figure 2-1) is represented in size, according to the number of times it appears. *Professional* is the largest word in the cloud, indicating its dominance in this document.

Among the explanations for the difficulty in conceptualizing and defining professionalism is the semantic one. The word *professional* is a broad overarching construct that serves as an umbrella for many related concepts that are each in themselves complex and abstract. Finding ways to measure some of the most abstract elements of *professional* have created a significant challenge for educators. One solution that occurs commonly is to omit difficult to measure concepts that are associated with professionalism. Anything that is abstract, subjective, or difficult to measure is extricated. For example, honorable or brave are rarely outcome measures in nursing education.

Figure 2-1   Word cloud of Essential VIII: Professionalism and Professional Values.*

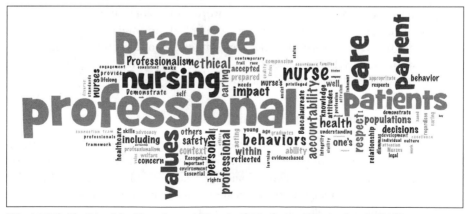

*The AACN's *The Essentials of Baccalaureate Education for Professional Nursing Practice* (2008).

The sharp distinction and clarity of meaning of professionalism has been lost through centuries of historical development and frequent use. Words generally lose their distinctiveness over time because they are used to reference things or ideas that were not part of the original meaning. The more a word is used to refer to additional situations or phenomena, the broader and more obscure the meaning of the word can become.

Cultural and political factors have contributed to relegating the word *professional* to its current broad and vague use. *Professional* has been freely applied to mean doing a good job, like having a carpet professionally cleaned. *Professional* is also used in a broader sense to label a person who is not a member of a distinct profession but someone who is expert or skilled at what he or she does. Another particularly detrimental use of professional is to describe an objective, impersonal manner, or, in some instances, an obsequious as Sartre's (1975) waiter in the café.

> His movement is quick and forward, . . . He comes toward the patrons with a step a little too quick. He bends forward a little too eagerly; his voice, his eyes express an interest a little too solicitous . . . (p. 314)

There are also misconceptions and myths about professionalism in the nursing literature. One such belief is that caring and professionalism are opposed and irreconcilable (Gardner, 1992; Ohlén & Segesten, 1998). Another is that professionals are more difficult to approach than other people and that professionals are elitist (Sullivan, 2005).

Multiple uses of a word represent what has aptly been called *meaning creep*. With meaning creep the meaning of a word can become so broad that one person's understanding of a word or phrase may be completely different from another's. The differences in understanding are like people speaking to each other in different languages. In other words, both language speakers mean the same thing but use different words, or use the same words to mean something entirely different. There is a semantic but not a substantive difference. At times, disagreements and misunderstandings are semantic rather than substantive and can be readily rectified once the inconsistency is identified.

Language use has a double effect. Using a word is diffusional and reduces its clarity for other language users through meaning creep but, at the same time, adds a richness to the word that is absent without use. *Professional* is a good example, in that, it has become a confusing yet central label of our discipline and other disciplines—not to mention the quality of the carpet cleaner's work.

The Two Paradigms of Professionalism

What does *professional* mean to nurse professionals and what does the word communicate? There are two major paradigms from which professionals and professionalism can be viewed: sociological and psychological (Barker, 1992; Begley, 2005; Pellegrino & Thomasma, 1993). Since the sociological or consensus paradigm is currently the dominant paradigm in professionalism, it is described first.

Sociological or Consensus Paradigm: The Doing

Professionalism, from the sociological paradigm, is set within a culture of professionals whose members hold a shared belief of how a professional is expected to practice a profession. The profession bestows membership to a professional and the professional is expected to follow the codes, duties, obligations, and responsibilities that are required by society and the profession. The ethical professional is merely instrumental in *doing* what is right, or moral. The consensus paradigm represents a legalistic understanding of professional and addresses behavior, not the nurse professional as an individual. The consensus or sociological paradigm is closely aligned with principled and outcome-based ethical traditions.

There are two major arguments against using the consensus paradigm as the sole or even as the dominant view of professionalism. When professionals are only professionals through social context, they become uniforms with nothing inside. That is, nurse professionals do what is expected by societal standards, but nothing in their individual character contributes to their professionalism. If, however, professionals are professionals only because they do what is expected by the society, then the problem of integrity arises. If the professional is only a social construct, then there is no restraining force to keep the professional honest. What does a professional do when no one is watching? What keeps the nurse honest? Will the nurse professional report a mistake if he or she can cover it up and no one will know?

The problem of an ethic based on social expectations is illustrated by the mythical story of the Ring of Gyges. The problem of the Ring of Gyges was brought to the attention of Socrates by an Athenian citizen. According to Plato's (1984/384–322 BC), account, the ring was magical; anyone who placed it upon his finger and manipulated in a specific way could become invisible. A shepherd found the ring, discovered its magical secret, and used it to seduce a queen, kill the rightful king, and take over a kingdom.

The Athenian citizen challenged Socrates to explain the reason why any person who could gain power or wealth through unethical acts and who was assured of not being discovered would not do the same. Socrates answered the challenge by claiming that injustice or outcomes never bring true happiness. Only good character and behaviors will do that. A person refrains from doing immoral things because of his or her nature and desire to do good. The Ring of Gyges illustrates the primacy of the psychological or individual dimension of ethics, which is in turn the primary paradigm of professionalism.

As the story of the Ring of Gyges demonstrates, the two paradigms are inherent in the wood and mortar of ethics—they are as pervasive as air, they are malleable but indestructible. Table 2-1 offers a simplified heuristic that contrasts each of the paradigms. These paradigms are called by different names but semantic differences do not replace substantive ones.

Table 2-1   Contrast of Sociological and Psychological Paradigms of Professionalism

Category	Sociological paradigm	Psychological paradigm
Overarching question	What do others expect of me?	How should I live as a professional?
Motivation	Externally driven	Internally driven
Education	Follow rules; consider benefits and risks; analysis and decision-making methods essential	Method to respond appropriately to situations; self-reflection essential
Goal	Meet role expectations	Live up to personal and professional ideal
Dealing with error/moral wrongdoing	Accept responsibility but only within context of a system error; less likely to frame error as personal shortcomings	Accept responsibility for error and integrate vulnerability as part of and reason for professional and personal growth
Timing of ethical choices/behavior	Meet ethical expectations when playing the role of the professional; compartmentalization of personal and professional life	Meet ethical expectations; ethical is ingrained and not compartmentalized
Primary identity	Instrumental and primarily of doing; achievement and work	Personal identity and primarily of being; achievement and work set within context of identity
Process	Transactional	Transformational

A sociological view of professionalism suggests that the individual is an individual only as the person relates to others. A person's life is compartmentalized into a number of roles that he or she assumes, like parent, child, nurse, or friend (Martin, 1999). For example, Nurse B is abusive to her children and cheats on financial matters and on her husband. Nurse B has excellent reviews at work and plays the role of the good nurse. In the sociological view, compartmentalizing personhood into roles leaves most readers sensing that this view lacks integrity. There is a strong sense for most of us, to quote William James (1975), that a purely socially constructed paradigm of professionalism is like an apple with a "worm at the core" (p. 121).

Kohlberg's (1968) theory of moral development coincides with the two paradigms and appears to be the motive behind conformity of moral agents. In the first four levels of lesser developed moral agency, people are motivated to avoid punishment, gain rewards, or gain approval. Conformity at the higher two levels are mediated through an imaginary ideal, impartial spectator or through self-assessment and personal condemnation. It appears that the ability for a person to internalize moral sensitivity and, critically, self-reflect on one's actions rather than to respond out of a socially constructed sense of morality reflects a higher level of moral functioning.

Dispensational or Psychological Paradigm: The Being

The psychological paradigm asserts that a professional is not merely outward behavior, not merely doing. A professional's behavior is more importantly the manifestation of a good personal moral life and of *being* a person who will make moral choices based on good character. The professional is viewed in total, as a whole person who lives a life where one strives to be a good person and professional who does good work.

The dispensational or psychological paradigm explains why a professional is someone who does the right thing even if no one is looking. Decisions and actions come from within, from a partially inherent and partially developed proclivity to do what is good. The arguments against this paradigm are the same as the argument against the virtue ethic tradition. There is no way to standardize and objectify what is meant by good or by the qualities that make one so. Second, the psychological paradigm places more responsibility for choices and actions on the individual. With the sociological paradigm, people's internal individuated world is separated from their social roles and actions.

Personal Identity

According to Yam (2004), personal identity also corresponds to these two paradigms: the social ideals and expectations of the discipline and the public and the personal, or inward, individual ideal and expectation. There may be problems when the disparity between the two results in professional and practice problems; for example, when a nurse provides care that is judged adequate by professional standards and ideals but not by the individual nurse's ideals of a good nurse. Nurse J gives a medication after calculating the dosage and rechecking the medication six rights three times; this is standard care in the United States. Nurse J has particular concerns about making a mistake and asks another nurse to recheck her calculations. This is an expression of Nurse J's personal professional standard of care or ideal. In being more careful to avoid error, she goes beyond the standard expected of the average nurse. In the same way, perception differences in the personal standard or ideal of care or professional behavior can be lower than what might be expected by the discipline. In such cases, poor care can be the result of discrepancy of perceptions. This disconnect between the public's and the discipline's ideal of care and one's individual ideal of care may explain, in part, why some nurses provide poor care and are unaware of a need for improvement.

Relating the Two Paradigms

What is the relationship between the two paradigms of professionalism? Disparate or dialectic? Contrary or complementary? Liaschenko and Peter (2004) called for a new ethic of professionalism that eliminates the older traditional ways and use of the words *profession* and *practice* altogether. The use of *profession* is criticized because of its use of moral theory based on principled theory and codes. On the other hand, practice is, they claim, too abstract: "nursing primarily as a practice is too elitist and morally superior" (p. 493). Both of these words and conceptualizations, Liaschenko and Peter believe, fail to respond to the moral challenges of contemporary health care and its multiple and complex relationships. Liaschenko and Peter advocate using the word *work* as the professional medium through which autonomy will be evident and that this autonomy will not be a sterile control but rather relational.

Liaschenko and Peter (2004) identified significant problems that arise in the nursing profession if we understand *professional* only as behaviors. However, they ignore the very aspect of professional—the individual character and virtues—that rescues the incomplete conceptualization of professionalism from being understood as only the consensus paradigm. The word *work* and the problems that limit its usefulness because it refers to a product and cannot carry the heavy load that has traditionally been borne by the word *professional*. We believe that Liaschenko and Peter are similar to many nurse scholars and ethicists who have an uncomfortable sense about our current use of and education in professionalism. But we also believe that they and others have dismissed professionalism because no inclusive view of professionalism that includes both paradigms has clearly been articulated in the nursing literature.

Perhaps the relationship between the two paradigms is best expressed as *essential* and *instrumental*. The personal psychological constitution of the nurse professional is essential to and the center or core of what it means to be a nurse professional. The inner moral life of individuals is the essence of who they are. The consensus paradigm serves as the means or instrument by which one's core individual professionalism is manifest, connecting the groups and relationships and bringing about the outward demonstration of the inner moral life of the individual. The essential, the inner moral life, and the virtues of one's character are the essence of professionalism.

THE MISSING EDUCATIONAL PIECE: ATTENDING TO THE PSYCHOLOGICAL AND ETHICAL SELF

Even though, the word *professional* is used extensively but it is given minimal attention by nurse educators and nurses in general in the *explicit* curricula. Nursing education focuses on competency in knowledge and psychomotor skill and strives to demonstrate learning through measurable changes. Competition for inclusion of additional areas of study is fierce, and the areas that are important are taught but may not be viewed as important as competency-related areas.

Professionalism and professional ethics is sometimes mistakenly thought to be addressed if other areas of ethics are taught. Ethics education in the healthcare professions, according to Rhodes and Cohen (2002), falls into two distinct groups: *applied bioethics* and *professional ethics*. Bioethics emerged as a subgroup of ethics in the 1960s (Stevens, 2001). The central concerns of bioethics are technology and patient-related ethical issues whereas professional ethics addresses the social and personal moral commitments of professionals (Stevens). Bioethics generally addresses topics like informed consent, end-of-life decisions, the moral appropriateness of fetal stem cell use in medicine, or issues of justice in healthcare distribution. Professional ethics developed as a subgroup of ethics at about the same time as bioethics and became a more prominent part of the ethical landscape to address difficult questions posed by professionals about their practice as professionals (Barker, 1992). Professional ethics is concerned with issues that relate to the professional character and behavior of the nurse, such as being truthful, engaging in conflicts of interest, being able to reject assignments, or transparency. Many of the topics may be related to bioethics or ethics but it is clear that a professional ethic, or the ethic of being a good professional, is different and only indirectly addressed in bioethics and traditional ethics courses (Rhodes & Cohen).

Some schools offer electives, or include as required courses, on professionalism or socialization to the profession, and in these programs the ethic of professionalism is included but the areas of concentration are the reteaching of moral theory and bioethics. Conceptualization of moral behavior by Rest (1986) may also help to illustrate the relationship of morality and professionalism. Rest divided morality into four distinct components: moral judgment, moral sensitivity, moral values or motivation, and moral character. Clearly bioethics and ethics in general as presented today address mainly the first two, making the values and character part of implicit curriculum.

Nursing students are often expected to develop the internal character of an ethical professional on their own or through implicit or hidden curriculum. If professionalism and professional ethics are taught explicitly, the focus is relegated to the social paradigm of role model exposure, knowledge of codes, and following rules.

The significance of the internalization of good character and professional ethic education were marginalized in nursing curricula. Thus, the stage was set for bioethics and the sociological paradigm to dominate nursing education. The psychological paradigm and virtue-based ethics took a back seat or, in some cases, were not even allowed on the bus.

SOCIOLOGICAL AND EDUCATIONAL FACTORS THAT CONTRIBUTE TO THE MISSING PIECE

There are reasons for the hollow state of professionalism in nursing education and in professional education in other disciplines as well. In the early to mid-20th century, the tradition of empiricism that had been part of the epistemological debate as a source of knowledge for centuries (Ayer, 1952), became highly dominant in many aspects of scholarly thought. Empiricism took the form of what was called *logical positivism* and devalued things or phenomenon that could not be empirically measured. This distilled empirical view bled into all areas of knowledge, science, and education. Nonempirical moral characteristics, like integrity, humility, and compassion, are not measurable and, therefore, simply nonexistent and certainly could not be taught.

The emphasis on empiricism set up the lopsided teaching of professionalism to include only the social and legal requirements set by a society (laws, codes, and standards). Secularization, among other social and political forces in the United States, has resulted in the removal of traditional religious thought from public discourse (Neuhaus, 1984). Reference to God or faith-based ideology ended discourse rather than contributed to it. Virtues, in a long-standing tradition from classical Greek and early Christian thought, characterize traits that, in today's climate, are often considered inappropriate and judgmental in a pluralistic, multicultural setting, particularly in the United States. Virtue ethics and religion are areas of discourse that often fall beyond the boundaries of acceptable discourse.

The quest for what might be called the vanishing, individually constructed professional raised concern for many disciplines, like medicine, law, and engineering (Bottery, 1995; Cherry, 2003; Harris, 2008; Pellegrino, 2002). For example, in medicine, the governing educational bodies, the Association of American Medical Colleges and the Accrediting Council for Graduate Medical Education, have launched major educational initiatives to enhance professional education in medical schools (Coulehan et al., 2003). The face of medical education is radically changing with a push to develop and measure professionalism in medical students in order to educate professional physicians (Papadakis et al., 2005).

REVISITING PROFESSIONALISM IN NURSING EDUCATION

As in other disciplines, progress in the profession hinges on the ability of the profession to critically evaluate nursing education and practice and to reestablish a view of professionals that includes the internally motivated professional who strives to live a life of excellence. We are poised as a discipline to explore a reemergence of the individual into moral and professional life. Professionalism in nursing has traditionally embodied the heart, mind, and soul of nursing and, if properly understood and articulated, can continue to provide a robust basis of professional nursing that is capable of guiding education and practice. If professionalism is properly understood, valued, and applied, faculty may educate students more explicitly and intentionally to become nurse professionals.

REFERENCES

American Association of Colleges of Nursing. (2008). *The essentials of baccalaureate education for professional nursing practice.* Washington, DC: Author.

Ayer, A. J. (1952). *Language, truth and logic.* New York: Dover Publications, Inc.

Barker, S. F. (1992). What is a profession? *Professional Ethics, 1*(1–2), 73–99.

Begley, A. M. (2005). Practicing virtue: A challenge to the view that a virtue centered approach to ethics lacks practical content. *Nursing Ethics, 12*(6), 622–637.

Bottery, M. (1995). Toward a concept of the ethical professional. *Professional Ethics, 4*(1), 23–48.

Chadwick, R., & Thompson, A. (2000). Professional ethics and labor disputes: Medicine and nursing in the United Kingdom. *Cambridge Quarterly of Healthcare, 9,* 483–497.

Cherry, M. J. (2003). Scientific excellence, professional virtue and the profit motive: The market and healthcare reform. *Journal of Medicine and Philosophy, 28*(3), 259–280.

Conrad, P. (2007). *The medicalization of society.* Baltimore: Johns Hopkins University Press.

Coulehan, J., Williams, P. C., McCreary, V., & Belling, C. (2003). The best lack all conviction: Biomedical ethics, professionalism, and social responsibilities. *Cambridge Quarterly of Healthcare Ethics, 12,* 21–38.

Crigger, N. (2005). Two models of mistake making in professional practice: Moving out of the closet. *Nursing Philosophy, 6,* 11–18.

Davis, M. (2001). Introduction. In M. Davis & A. Stark (Eds.), *Conflict of interest in the professions* (pp. 1–19). Oxford, UK: Oxford University Press.

Ford, J. (2008). Annual legislative update. A state-by-state report. *ADVANCE for Nurse Practitioners, 16*(12), 51–52.

Gardner, K. (1992). The historical conflict between caring and professionalization: A dilemma for nursing. In D. A. Gaut (Ed.), *The presence of caring in nursing* (pp. 241–255). New York: National League for Nursing.

Harris, C. E. (2008). The good engineer: Giving virtue its due in engineering ethics. *Science Engineering Ethics, 14*(2), 153–164.

James, W. (1975). *The varieties of religious experience.* New York: Mentor Book.

Klein, T. (2008). Credentialing the nurse practitioner in your workplace. *Nursing Administration Quarterly, 32*(4), 273–276.

Kohlberg, L. (1968). The child as moral philosopher. *Psychology Today, 7,* 25–30.

Liaschenko, J., & Peter, E. (2004). Nursing ethics and conceptualizations of nursing: Profession, practice and work. *Journal of Advanced Nursing, 46*(5), 488–495.

Luebke, N. R. (1989). Conflict of interest as a moral category. *Business & Professional Ethics Journal, 6*(1), 66–81.

Martin, M. (1999). Explaining wrongdoing in professions. *Journal of Social Philosophy, 30*(2), 236–250.

Neuhaus, R. J. (1984). *The naked public square.* Grand Rapids, MI: Eerdmans.

Ohlén, J., & Segesten, K. (1998). The professional identity of the nurse: Concept analysis and development. *Journal of Advanced Nursing, 28*(4), 720–727.

Papadakis, M. A., Teherani, A., Banach, M. A., Knettler, T. R., Rattner, S. L., Stern, D. T., et al. (2005). Disciplinary action by medical boards and prior behavior in medical school. *The New England Journal of Medicine, 353,* 2673–2682.

Pellegrino, E. D. (2002). Rationing health care: Inherent conflicts within the concept of justice. In W. B. Bondeson & J. W. Jones (Eds.), *The ethics of managed care: profession integrity and patient rights* (pp. 1–18). Dordrecht, The Netherlands: Kluwer Academic Publishers.

Pellegrino, E. D., & Thomasma, D. C. (1993). *The virtues in medical practice.* New York: Oxford University Press.

Plato. (1984). *The Republic, Book II, 360* (2nd ed., D. Lee, Trans.). New York: Penguin Books. (Original work published 384–322 BC)

Rest, J. R. (1986). *Moral development: Advances in research and theory.* New York: Praeger.

Rhodes, R., & Cohen, R. (2002). Two concepts of medical ethics and their implications for medical education. *Journal of Medicine and Philosophy, 27*(4), 493–508.

Sartre, J. P. (1975). Sartre: Existentialism. In W. Kaufman (Ed.), *Existentialism: From Dostoevsky to Sartre* (pp. 280–374). New York: Meridian.

Stevens, T. (2001). *Bioethics in America: Origins and cultural politics.* Baltimore: Johns Hopkins University Press.

Sullivan, W. M. (2005). *Work and integrity* (2nd ed.). San Francisco: Jossey-Bass.

Yam, B. M. C. (2004). From vocation to profession: The quest for professionalization of nursing. *British Journal of Nursing, 13*(16), 978–982.

CHAPTER 3

Roots and Branches of Professionalism

Moral life flows from character—
ingrained, concrete, steady, like a second nature.

—LEON KASS, 2002

The authors could not evaluate nursing professionalism without a knowledge of the trends in professionalism of other disciplines. As with all disciplines, conceptualizing professionalism draws from both the general substantive elements of professionalism that are applicable to all disciplines and the elements that are specific to each discipline (Holm, 2006; Martin & Gabard, 2001). Exploring the nature of professionalism and what qualifies a discipline as a profession has only recently reemerged as a topic of interest in many disciplines. The sections of this chapter describe the historical, social, and linguistic development of professionalism and professions, and the factors that have brought us to the current understanding of professionalism in other professions and in nursing.

THE HISTORICAL AND SOCIAL ROOTS OF PROFESSIONS

Professionals and Ethical Commitment

Society grants special status to professionals but, in turn, professionals have obligations and duties to society and the discipline for the privilege of practicing their profession (Bottery, 2005; Pellegrino, 2005). Nurses' scope of practice in the United States delineates the services that society has granted the professional nurse to perform through legal licensure. In a society where no governmental licensure exists, degree granting institutions take the responsibility for sanctioning professional practice. For example, some developing nations rely on educational institutions to grant practice privileges rather than the legal process of governmental licensure. Honduras, for example, has no governmental body that is responsible for licensure; rather, the Universities are the institutions that grant practice privileges. In either case, once requirements and qualifications to become a professional member of a discipline are met, the individual is publicly acknowledged as a member of that discipline. The history of public acknowledgment as a prerequisite of formal admission to profession membership dates back to the traditions of scholastic institutions during the Middle Ages. New members of a profession "professed" their commitment to the profession.

27

Contemporary activities for a graduate or undergraduate degree continue to be similar to the Middle Ages in the sense of public acknowledgment and professional commitment through ceremonies, graduations, and awards. The graduate receives a diploma and is granted the rights, responsibilities, and privileges of this accomplishment by the degree-granting institution.

From Whence Professions Came

Historically, *profession* and *professionalism* were first used as descriptors in law, medicine, and the clergy. In medieval times, oaths and vows took on great meaning and tradition had a much deeper impact on society than it has during the modern and postmodern eras (Smith, 2001). The verb *profess* was originally Latin, passing into Middle English and French and meant to announce publicly (*Webster's New Universal Unabridged Dictionary*, 1989). According to Barker (1992), *profession* came into use in the late Middle Ages and was originally used to mean "proclaim" or "declare" but later came to refer to making to religious vows. Beginning in the 16th century, profession was used in the occupations, particularly medicine, and indicated the self-interest of the members of the discipline rather than as altruistic commitment to the people they served.

The French playwright Moliere wrote the *Imaginary Invalid*, a satire on physicians during the latter half of the 17th century. Moliere's spoof may have reflected the public view of physicians during his era. The mistrust of physicians ultimately led to a major reformation of the medical profession that brought about the higher moral consensus of integrity and altruistic commitment to the profession (Pellegrino & Thomasma, 1993).

Historical development of professions in the 20th century was marked by the emergence of a new economy after World War II that was characterized by the movement of the private sector into what was formerly the public sector (Bottery, 2005; Rothman & Rothman, 2003). Cherry (2003) described the impact on health care as the movement from the covenant or fiduciary role of the healthcare provider to one of the business contract. The concern of the replacement of traditional professionalism by entrepreneurship has resulted in a largely negative response from many different disciplines (Cherry; Pellegrino, 2005; Sullivan, 2005). According to Sullivan, the new economy may be a greater threat to professionalism than it is a benefit. The new workers and professionals have a stronger link to success and success is often linked to monetary return. "Innovation, efficacy and traveling light psychologically, with few loyalties" (Sullivan, p. 7) are the hallmarks of the new economy worker.

The 1980s to the present are marked by a new type of professional who is raised with a strong sense of personal freedom and an ability to instantaneously "get what we want" (Sullivan, 2005, p. 18). Communication, travel, and global access reinforce this instant gratification with society and professionals alike. Sullivan and others describe major social changes brought by so-called yuppies—persons characterized by a drive toward high levels of material security and self-fulfillment, a high degree of competitive pressure, and yet were fragmented in their personal and professional lives. Life and career became an effort toward winning and increasing power, with resulting emptiness. Sullivan explained that winning may plateau; if gratification and success rest only on winning, there is surely a problem. Loss and decline are a part of human existence; therefore, life becomes hollow if these particular values are the only ones individuals possess. These social, political, and legal changes have challenged the idea of professional such that professions and the group of individuals represented by it are in what Sullivan and others have termed a *crisis of professionalism.*

More recently, the erosion of public confidence has contributed to some disciplines becoming more concerned with their image. Efforts to improve the public image include more community involvement and awareness. A recently aired television advertisement produced by the American Medical Association shows a man jogging, saying that people's perception of heroes often does not include physicians. The actor-jogger tells the audience that his physician was a hero because the physician saved his life.

Work to improve a sagging public image is not limited to medicine (Kuczewski, Bading, Langbein, & Henry, 2003; Larkin, 2003). Lawyers (Rizzardi, 2005), accountants (Sullivan, 2005), educators (Bottery, 1995), public servants like police (Bottery, 1995), and journalists (Lichtenberg, 1989) are aware of the increased scrutiny by a more discerning public. Many have initiatives to improve their professional status among the public.

Business and Professionalism

The business model in health care and in the private sector has had a profound impact on public and professions views of professionalism (Conrad, 2007; Pellegrino & Thomasma, 1993). The conflation of the business model into the professional model has not been as sudden of a change as some might suspect, but rather began just after World War II and represents a slow and gradual shift toward adoption of the model (Rothman & Rothman, 2003).

Health care as a business, particularly in the United States, changes the way professionals and patients think about health care. Professionals are now providers, treatments are referred to as goods and services, and patients are consumers of these goods and services. Economy has become a driving force behind advancing biotechnology, health management, and resource utilization. Research, also impacted by business, is funded by private section special interest groups and conflict of interest becomes of greater concern as companies establish questionable ties with professional institutions and individuals (Angell, 2004). As Conrad (2007) claimed, innovation in the healthcare arena that was formerly motivated by knowledge acquisition has now become motivated by the market and social forces.

Despite the economic benefits of conjoining business with the traditional professionalism, ethically, the two are uneasy bedfellows and these differences have sparked significant public debate (Cherry, 2003; Sullivan, 2005). The topic is complex and the literature provides evidence that the blending of the two models has both positive and negative effects. Profiting from some aspects may be morally questionable and erode the public view of professionals (Crigger, Courter, Hamacher, Hayes, & Shepherd, 2009) but, at the same time, the addition of business may have empowered people with alternative choices and boosted productivity and creativity. The relationship of professionals with business is thought by many to set up problematic conflicts of interest that can result in immoral behavior by healthcare providers (Angell, 2004; Crigger, Junko, Rahal, Barnes, & Sheek, 2009), whereas in some circumstances business may improve provider productivity and increase provider knowledge. Business has been cast as the cause of institutionalized injustice, forgetting that business is the engine of economy and that business competition brings free market and creative solutions and reduces cost. At a risk of oversimplification, key elements of the business model and the traditional professional model gleaned from the literature are compared in Table 3-1.

Table 3-1   Contrast of Traditional Professionalism with Business

	Traditional professionalism model	Business model
Care decisions	Fiduciary; professional acts in best interest of the care recipient and the common good	Consumer-driven choice
Presentation to the care recipient	Burdens and benefits weighed objectively	Market creates need; burdens downplayed and benefits emphasized
Empowerment	Care recipient	External through obtaining goods and services
Strategy for care	Least expensive and intrusive	Expense equates with better care; newer equates with better care
Goal or outcome for professional	Personal professional identity and satisfaction	Produce and increase market share
Relation with society	Cooperative	Competitive

REFLECTIONS ON NURSE PROFESSIONALISM

The Busy Fragmented Nurse

Nurses, like many people in today's busy world, live fragmented lives and go about their work with limited time and energy to devote to the many immediacy of life and demands of family (Sullivan, 2005). The percentage of nurses who join professional organizations appears to have declined, along with support for the profession in general, or for alma maters. The waning of the professional culture is predictable, according to Sullivan and is evidence of change at two levels: larger society and the smaller personal ways in which people of contemporary society live their lives (Pellegrino & Thomasma, 1993).

Nurse M works an extra hour finishing paperwork at her job, drives the 20 minutes home, only to arise from 6 hours of sleep at 6 AM to shuttle her son to an out-of-town soccer game. The day is just beginning. Upon arriving home after the soccer game, Nurse M moves deftly and deliberately through her long "to do" list. She is a single parent and has no one else to help with household chores. Priorities are set and thoughts are task-oriented; there are many more goals that compete for completion than are completed. Things are crowded in, back-to-back. Life feels like a blur. "My life," she thinks, "is like cramming 5 pounds of potatoes into a 2-pound bag." Nurse M thinks about a lingering cup of coffee, a warm crackling fire, and just time to think. But not today. Nurse M is the norm rather than the exception and illustrates the frantic lifestyle that has increasingly become life in the 21st century.

Parallels can be drawn between contemporary society and the postwar German society that distressed Martin Heidegger (1956). Heidegger warned of the dangers of life lived in an increasingly technological society. Germans were more mobile, more engaged, and, he believed, too busy to live life authentically. There are, he claimed, two types of thinking: meditative and calculative. Meditative thinking is not marked by productivity and allows reflectiveness, whereas calculative thinking, although productive, is a *flight from thinking* (p. 45). Calculative thinking is, in reality, a thoughtlessness primarily because it limits meditative thinking. He wrote:

> All of us, including those who think professionally, . . . are often enough thought-poor, we are all too easily thought-less. (pp. 44–45)

> For nowadays we take in everything in the quickest and cheapest way, only to forget it just as quickly. (p. 45)

> But part of this flight is that man will neither see nor admit it. (p. 45)

People often take the flight from thinking while living everyday lives. Professional ethics and issues of professionalism are notoriously ambiguous, likely demanding Heidegger's (1956) meditative thought, and are time intensive. There is little time for the more fundamental and ultimate concerns of life and reflection. Days, even weeks go by, caught up in the day-to-day instrumental, calculative thinking. Although calcula-tive thinking serves particular purposes, too much can leave little time for meditative thinking. We are inculcations of our culture, and our culture is evidence based, out-come oriented, and market driven. Heidegger was distressed about the lack of medita-tive thinking believing it to be essential for society and, we add, for professionals in education and professional practice.

Another important psychological condition that has resulted from the modern social environment was identified and coined by Gergen (2001) as *multiphrenic*. Multiphrenic does not refer to a select few people with a psychiatric disorder but, rather, to many people who are living in contemporary globalized society. Multiphrenia is the fragmentation and decentering that results primarily from tech-nology being the method that brings large numbers of social contacts and information sources to an individual. The competing sources of information and relationships, and the multiplicity of conflicting information, result in disorientation, cynicism, and difficulty in decision making.

Quest for Identity

Nursing literature on professionalism has been limited. Of the existing journal arti-cles, publications on *professional identity* dominate the literature. First, is nursing a profession? The argument about entry into practice is thought to negatively impact the acceptance of nursing as a profession and may have shifted attention away from other important issues of professionalism (Girard, 2005; Joel, 2002; Keogh, 1997). The second question relates to the first and is a quest for knowledge, theories, and ethics that establish nursing's unique status and sets the discipline apart from all others (Liaschenko & Peter, 2004; Myhrvold, 2006; Naef, 2006).

As significant as activities to promote and establish a distinct identity might be, it has come with a price. Some of the efforts to individualize a discipline lead to isola-tion because, in claiming the uniqueness, we may reject the commonalities of prac-tice, ethics, and professionalism that are shared with other professions. For example, nursing diagnosis does not share the common language of diagnoses with other disci-plines. There is nothing adverse about seeking distinctive recognition for the discipline, but there may be something adverse if we fail to recognize a common inheritance and participation in ethics and professionalism. The nursing profession is affected by the same social influences that are devaluing professions and professionals elsewhere.

Nursing as a discipline is influenced but not driven exclusively by external forces of society. There is and should be a strong desire within the profession to establish who nurses are as professionals and as a profession, and to successfully avoid the crisis of professionalism that is currently impacting many other disciplines (Sullivan, 2005). The nursing discipline's struggle for legitimacy as a profession does not appear to negatively influence society's view of nurses. According to the average citizen's intuitive response, and to some professional ethics authorities such as Davis (2002) and Sullivan, nursing is a highly esteemed altruistic profession that is similar to teaching and social work (Joel, 2002).

As a discipline and a profession, nurses' primary responsibility is to a profession and to recipients of care: "a profession means that one declares herself as a member of a profession and conducts herself according to the profession's standards" (Davis, 2002, p. 48). Professionalism means "putting the client first when the profession claims that that is what [nurses] are supposed to do" (Davis, 2002, p. 48).

The relationship between the patient and the nurse is, first and foremost, an ethical one. Nurse professionals, like any other professional with a fiduciary relationship, practice with the focus on the best interest of the patient. The best interest of the patient differs from patient desire. The distinction between the business model and the professional fiduciary model, as addressed previously, is clear about the juncture of interest and desire. The business model gives a patient what he or she wants but the professional model attends to what is best for the patient. For example, a patient asks you, as a nurse practitioner, to provide her with a prescription refill. By refilling the prescription she will continue to delay a much needed follow-up visit to the prescribing doctor because of the cost for the visit. From a human perspective, you feel compassionate and your heart goes out to this individual. Yet, as a professional, you know that the follow-up care is in her best interest, so you say no. Some feminist theory may challenge this conclusion and perhaps with good justification. However, if the best interest is served, clearly the patient's desire should be acknowledged but, as a professional, the nurse's moral commitment is to the patient's best interests.

THE LINGUISTIC ROOTS OF PROFESSIONS AND PROFESSIONALS

Etymological Understanding

Professions and professionals who are members of the profession are empowered by society and are called to higher moral standards than are the general public. They are responsible for upholding key public values and performing specialized service (Sullivan, 2005). Yet these words, no matter how significant, have another quality common to many words; they become slippery when we try to establish clarity and exactness of what they are. When we define profession or professionals, we are forced, as Davis (2002) claimed, to make a "choice between the important and the incidental" (p. 1). If words are swords, then the choice of how to use them is the powerful swing of the sword. For example, are there professional strippers? Can we claim that the waiter, by his or her impersonal but attentive service, is acting like a professional?

Words are more than definitions and uses; they are living and dynamic reflections of the society in which they exist and, at the same time, shaping the society. Words are born, they grow through use by language speakers, and they transform. Words may even die. Word graveyards are full of words or uses of words that are long dead. Hail no longer means hello, and prithee, which meant please in Shakespeare's time, is no longer used. The understanding of the meanings and uses of words is in itself a complex undertaking. Our inquiry into *profession* and *professionals*, in order to be thorough, first begins in the etymological and historical life of the word *profession* from which *professional*, the individual human unit, is derived.

As noted previously, a word has two aspects to consider: its meaning and its use. In some ways, words are like generic and trade names. There is one generic or meaning but there may be multiple trade names or uses. Unlike generic and trade names, meaning and use of words have a transforming relationship with each other.

The words *profession* and *professional* have a historical development of uses or senses that broaden understanding of the words and, in turn, impact meaning. When we say a word, it likely has shared uses: ones for which a consensus can be obtained and specific uses that may be for as small a consensus of two. For example, twins or an intimate couple may invent words or use established words in ways that are shared only between the two people.

Professions and *professionals* can also be used directly and indirectly. *Denotation* is the direct referent to an object(s) or phenomenon(a) and *connotation* involves indirect associations that are expressed by use of a word. Both denotation and connotation have shared uses, yet can also be widely diverse. Denotation of some object or phenomenon is a metaphorical finger pointing at a referent. For example, rug denotes a carpet throughout a house but also a bear rug by the fireplace. Both are rugs, but both have very different qualities. Connotation of words can be even more obscure. Connotations are like spiders in a web and speak to the vast connections and associations that words have. Word are embedded and connected to many other words and ideas. Speakers can use the word *caring*, for example, and relate caring to their perception of mothers by their role, kittens by their being the object of affection, or thoughtful actions, like birthday gifts. Another person may find caring indicative of the tough love of leaving a child in jail overnight or of making a bed as an act of service.

There are many levels of cultural consensus for word usage. Used within disciplines or community of consensus words also have generally applicable uses as well as uses that are highly specific to the discipline. For example, consider the word *random*. In ordinary or common language, if random is used to describe how we select people for a group, it refers to a haphazard method of choice. However, random in research means specifically that the selection is systematic and allows for select from the group to be representative. In teaching, research students often fail to see the distinction between ordinary use and its specific use in research.

Often, a true account of the word goes back to its origin. The word *profession* is rooted in Latin *professios* that meant to avow publicly. Later the French and Middle

English meaning of the word was to make a vow publicly, and even later to make a vow publicly that indicated commitment to a profession or group and to service (Barker, 1992).

Related Words and Concepts

A number of words relate to *professional*, *professionalism*, and *profession* that have been used and, in some instances, are better suited to address what nursing is and does. Van Hooft (2006) used the metaphor of family. Words that relate and can be used similarly are like family members' relationship to each other. Sometimes using another word may be beneficial but may also confound a distinct and clear understanding of a word. Ambiguity of language is the rule rather than exception and is in part responsible for our discipline's wide and current use of conceptual analyses.

The source of words, the traditional meaning, helps to explicate their use. Synonyms are words that have the same or similar meaning in one or more senses. Synonyms are not exactly the same as another word, but can be used in some situations to reference the same idea or thing. There are several family members to consider in the case of professionalism. *Occupation* originates from a Latin word that means to possess or to employ. The understanding is that one is occupied by work. A profession is an occupation, but not all occupations are professions.

Vocation is understood as the business of one's life that comes from a Latin word that means to call or summon. Implicit in vocation is the idea that the individual has been *called* into the profession. Vocation was originally applied to the ministry. In some circumstances, a person of religious or humanitarian might feel that God's providence has brought them to engage in a certain vocation; thus, some people see nursing as a vocation whereas others do not. White (2002) has suggested that vocation is better suited to address nursing and elevates nursing to a higher order than does profession.

Work is also used by some language speakers as the defining feature that addresses nursing's response to today's social realities (Liaschenko & Peter, 2004). Liascheko and Peter (2004) advocate work to best describe nursing because that is what nurses do. The word *work* means to labor, toil, or produce. Nursing is certainly work, but so is construction work and food service work. There is nothing in the word that marks distinction from other forms of labor.

Job is akin to *work* and originally referred to a glob in the mouth. Then, a job became the shorter term for *work* and is most analogous to a task or piece of work that is limited in time and scope.

The term *career* originates from Middle English and French and means a road or race course. In one sense, professionals may change their profession or work one time or more. Professionals may drop out of professional roles altogether or may have started their lives working as nonprofessionals. The course of life work becomes a career, and the word inherently means something over time—a lifetime—that may or may not involve professional work.

The last word, *competency* has been used in nursing since the 1990s, and is particularly favored in nursing education and is most commonly defined as "the ability to perform a job or occupation" (Axley, 2008, p. 216; *Webster's New Universal Unabridged Dictionary*, 1985). Historically the use of competency in nursing was limited to technical function but appears to have been used in a more expansive way to include insight, psychological attitudes, and motives (Axley).

Is a competent nurse also a professional nurse? Can these terms be interchanged? There are two differences that suggest that the term is not synonymous in most uses. Competency indicates that one has acquired sufficiency in the ability to perform a job. The competent nurse is not indicating a measure of quality but rather of safety, what is needed to be minimally prepared to do the work. As a beginning nurse professional, competency should be the goal, but certainly not as the nurse continues along the path of a professional life. Nurse educators' goals are to educate nurses to grow beyond sufficiency and safety to become good or excellent.

Competency is the ability or potential not yet applied to situations. Work by Edmondson and Pearce (2006) make the case for the use of *wisdom*, a word used for millennia, to address application of knowledge to real world practice. They argue that one can have capacity and knowledge without actually participating in real-life situations. The student with competency in skills and a good knowledge base but who is inadequate in clinical settings that require application is familiar to most educators. The conception of wisdom as application comes close to the Aristotelean ideal of practical wisdom, or phronesis.

In review, many words have similar meanings and can be used synonymously with professional in some senses, but the words *profession* and *professional* are very distinct terms with a rich historical development. None of these words that are at times substituted for *profession* and *professional* mean the same thing in all senses. Therefore, the synonyms and closely related words cannot do the same work as *profession* and *professionalism*. To replace these words would deny the significant historical heritage of *professions* and *professionalism* and its distinct meaning.

PROFESSIONS DEFINED

In view of the historical development of professions, it is no surprise that there is no one source that identifies all of the critical elements of a profession. Reliable sources in and outside of nursing can be synthesized to construct a view of the nursing profession. Four different sources were used to evaluate the characteristics of a profession (Table 3-2). A landmark work describing the characteristics of a profession was offered by Flexner nearly 100 years ago (Killeen & Saewert, 2007) and gave a historical perspective to professions. Flexner identified professional personal qualities more

Table 3-2 Defining Characteristics of a Profession

Area of comparison	Flexner (1910)*	Battin (1990)	Davis (2002)	Nursing
Social structure	Strong internal organization	Distinct group who provides service to a specific group of recipients	Defined collaborative group	
Economics		Fee for service	Fee for service	
Professional ethics		Has a group acceptance of rules, regulates or codes that govern; expectation that the practitioner is loyal to the profession	Consensus of what moral professional is; establishes codes and standards, and member chooses to accept them; held to higher standard of morality than nonmembers	Responsibility of members to expand knowledge in discipline (Keogh, 1997); special calling (Girard, 2005)
Body of knowledge		Specialized body of knowledge		Specialized body of knowledge (Killeen & Saewert, 2007); knowledge is acquired through research (Keogh, 1997; Killeen & Saewert, 2007)

(continues)

Table 3-2 Defining Characteristics of a Profession (*continued*)

Area of comparison	Flexner (1910)*	Battin (1990)	Davis (2002)	Nursing
Education	Can be taught	Extended period of formal education		Prolonged education in university (Killeen & Saewert, 2007)
Government regulation and benefits		Licensure or credentialing	Monopoly on services through licensure	
Self-governing		Self-regulatory/discipline in place; public acknowledgment as a group		Autonomous in decision making (Killeen & Saewert, 2007)
Relation to recipients of care		Inequality of power with recipient of care		
Altruism and service	Practitioners are altruistic			Service orientation (Joel, 2002)
Autonomy in practice	High responsibility in practice			Autonomy of practice (Gerrish et al., 2003)
Work	Basically intellectual; practical not theoretical			

*As reported by Killeen and Saewert, 2007.

than any of the other sources, claiming that the member of a profession was altruistic, learned, responsible, and used practical application.

Michael Davis (2002), a well-known professional ethicist and advocate of the consensus paradigm (although he does not use this term), believes that professions are defined as "a number of individuals in the same occupation who voluntarily organized to earn a living by openly serving in a morally-permissible way beyond what (ordinary) morality would require" (p. 3). He believes that the social paradigm of following the rules is enough for one to be a member of a profession. Davis believes this definition to be the best practical clarification. His view of professions differs from the others in that members charge a fee for service is a critical element of a profession.

Margaret Battin (1990), another well-known philosopher, developed a list of 13 characteristics of professions that emerged from a literature review. Battin's characteristics are more precise than Davis' but both appear to be consistent, aside from Davis' implicit reference to education and credentialing through following the profession's expectations and rules.

From a nursing perspective, Joel (2002) describes three common areas of agreement in nursing: service orientation, autonomous agency, and that the profession is learned through education. Yet, the areas of agreement as described by Joel seem limited when compared to the previously discussed characteristics expressed by Davis or Battin. Additional characteristics that have emerged from the literature include Gerrish, McManus, and Ashworth's (2003) use of autonomy, privilege, and power as a defining characteristics. Keogh (1997) added research and the idea of expanding knowledge as a part of professionalism. Fetzer (2003) claimed that nurses have a special calling into the profession, whereas Girard (2005) takes education into the university setting as a defining characteristic of professionals. The two most agreed-upon characteristics appear to be the social nature of the organization and its strong member expectations that are formalized in rules, codes, or standards. Interestingly, Killeen and Saewert (2007) report that the most common defining characteristics of the nursing profession are a specialized body of knowledge and altruism. From the review of the four sources in Table 3-2, the most common characteristics and that appear most consistently are education and the strong social expectations expressed as codes and standards.

DEFINING PROFESSIONALISM IN NURSING

We now turn from *professions* to *professional*. The professional is an individual who properly uses internal resources of the self to meet social expectations and personal ideals.

As nurse ethicists, the authors distinguish between *nurse professional* and *professional nurse*. By nurse professional we mean a person who professes to be a member of the discipline and has individual characteristics that inform and motivate him or her to make good moral choices. A nurse professional becomes a professional nurse through validation by education and examination or by institutional verification.

HEGEMONY IN NURSING, ETHICS, AND PROFESSIONALISM

With closer scrutiny of ethics and professionalism, a clearer relationship is emerging. Professionalism across disciplines and in nursing is deeply connected to the ethic within the discipline and within individual nurse professionals. Within the discipline of nursing, growing pains regarding professionalism and ethics are evident. A deeper understanding of both concepts is needed so that nurse professionals can more clearly articulate what it means to reflect excellence in character and practice. Ethics in nursing has been characterized in a struggle between what is unique to nursing and what is common to all professionals and ethically relevant situations (Myhrvold, 2006; Naef, 2006; Scott, 2006). Surprisingly, both can be addressed through an inclusive framework, a solution that has also been suggested as an alternative for nursing ethics (McCarthy, 2006).

REFERENCES

Angell, M. (2004). *The truth about drug companies: How they deceive what and us to do about it.* New York: Random House.

Axley, L. (2008). Competency: A concept analysis. *Nursing Forum, 43*(4), 214–222.

Barker, S. F. (1992). What is a profession? *Professional Ethics, 1*(1–2), 73–99.

Battin, M. (1990). *Ethics in the sanctuary.* New Haven, CT: Yale University Press.

Bottery, M. (1995). Toward a concept of the ethical professional. *Professional Ethics, 4*(1), 23–47.

Bottery, M. (2005). The individualization of consumption, educational management. *Administration & Leadership, 33*(3), 267–288.

Cherry, M. J. (2003). Scientific excellence, professional virtue and the profit motive: The market and healthcare reform. *Journal of Medicine and Philosophy, 28*(3), 259–280.

Conrad, P. (2007). *The medicalization of society.* Baltimore: Johns Hopkins University Press.

Crigger, N., Courter, L., Hamacher, M., Hayes, K., & Shepherd, K. (2009). Public perceptions of healthcare participation in pharmaceutical marketing. *Nursing Ethics, 16*(5), 647–658.

Crigger, N., Junko, A., Rahal, S., Barnes, K., & Sheek, C. (2009). Nurse practitioners' perceptions of pharmaceutical marketing and conflict of interests. *Journal of Advanced Nursing, 65*(3), 125–133.

Davis, M. (2002). *Profession, code and ethics: Toward a morally useful theory of today's professions.* Hants, England: Ashgate Publishing Limited.

Edmondson, R., & Pearce, J. (2006). The practice of health care: Wisdom as a model. *Medicine, Health Care and Philosophy, 10*, 233–244.

Fetzer, S. J. (2003). Professionalism of associate degree nurses: The role of socialization. *Nursing Education Perspectives*, *24*(3), 139–143.

Gergen, K. (2001). *The saturated self: Dilemmas of identity in contemporary life* (2nd ed.). New York: Basic Books.

Gerrish, K., McManus, M., & Ashworth, P. (2003). Creating what sort of professional? Master's level nurse education as a professionalising strategy. *Nursing Inquiry*, *10*(2), 103–112.

Girard, N. J. (2005). Are you a professional? *AORN Journal*, *81*(3), 487–488.

Heidegger, M. (1956). *Discourse on thinking*. Translated by J. M. Anderson & E. H. Freund. New York: Harper & Row.

Holm, S. (2006). What should other healthcare professions learn from nursing ethics. *Nursing Philosophy*, *7*, 165–174.

Joel, L. A. (2002). Education for entry into nursing practice: Revisited for the 21st century. *The Online Journal of Issues in Nursing*, *7*(2). Available at: http://www.nursingworld.org/ojin/topic18/tpc18_4.htm

Keogh, J. (1997). Professionalization of nursing: development, difficulties and solutions. *Journal of Advanced Nursing*, *25*, 302–308.

Killeen, M. L., & Saewert, L. J. (2007). Socialization to professional nursing. In J. L. Creasia & B. J. Parker (Eds.), *Conceptual foundations: The bridge to professional nursing practice* (pp. 49–80). St. Louis, MO: Mosby Elsevier.

Kuczewski, M. G., Bading, E., Langbein, M., & Henry, B. (2003). Fostering professionalism: The Loyola Model. *Cambridge Quarterly of Healthcare Ethics*, *12*, 161–166.

Larkin, G. L. (2003). Mapping, modeling, and mentoring: Charting a course for professionalism in graduate medical education. *Cambridge Quarterly of Healthcare Ethics*, *12*, 167–177.

Liaschenko, J., & Peter, E. (2004). Nursing ethics and conceptualizations of nursing: Profession, practice and work. *Journal of Advanced Nursing*, *46*(5), 488–495.

Lichtenberg, J. (1989). Truth, neutrality, and conflict of interest. *Business & Professional Ethics Journal*, *9*(1–2), 65–78.

McCarthy, J. (2006). A pluralist view of nursing ethics. *Nursing Philosophy*, *7*, 157–164.

Martin, M. W., & Gabard, D. L. (2001). Conflict of interest and physical therapy. In M. Davis & A. Stark (Eds.), *Conflict of interest in the professions* (pp. 314–332). Oxford, UK: Oxford University Press.

Myhrvold, T. (2006). The different other-towards an including ethic of care. *Nursing Philosophy*, *7*, 125–136.

Naef, R. (2006). Bearing witness: A moral way of engaging in the nurse-person relationship. *Nursing Philosophy*, *7*, 146–156.

Pellegrino, E. D. (2005). Professionalism, profession and the virtues of the good physician. *The Mount Sinai Journal of Medicine*, *69*(6), 378–384.

Pellegrino, E. D., & Thomasma, D. C. (1993). *The virtues in medical practice*. New York: Oxford University Press.

Rizzardi, K. W. (2005). Defining professionalism, I know it when I see it? *The Florida Bar Journal*, *July/August*, 38–43.

Rothman, S. M., & Rothman, D. J. (2003). *The pursuit of perfection*. New York: Random House.

Scott, P. A. (2006). Perceiving the moral dimension of practice: Insights from Murdoch, Vetlesen and Aristotle. *Nursing Ethics, 7*, 137–145.

Smith, H. (2001). *Why religion matters: The fate of the human spirit in an age of disbelief*. New York: HarperCollins

Sullivan, W. M. (2005). *Work and integrity* (2nd ed.). San Francisco: Jossey-Bass.

Webster's new universal unabridged dictionary (2nd ed.). (1985). New York: Simon & Schuster.

Van Hooft, S. (2006). *Understanding virtue ethics*. Chesham, UK: Acumen Publishing Limited.

White, K. (2002). Nursing as vocation. *Nursing Ethics, 9*(3), 279–290.

SECTION 2

Is It Possible to Develop an Inclusive Ethical Framework for Nurse Professionals?

CHAPTER 4

The Place of Virtue Ethics Within Nursing

[T]here is a telos which transcends
the limited goods of practices by constituting
the good of a whole human life.

—MacIntyre, 1984

Just as the individual vanished from professional discussion, virtue ethics was marginalized for decades while deontological and consequential ethical traditions dominated the ethical landscape. In recent years, scholars, ethicists, and theorists from other disciplines and a number of nursing ethicists outside the United States have been part of the renewed interest in virtue ethics. Because virtue ethics tradition is complex and has often been misinterpreted and applied in a variety of ways (Hursthouse, 2009), the authors describe the Greek traditions of virtue ethics and, to a lesser extent, the virtue tradition that is embedded in the Eastern intellectual thought of Confucianism. Using MacIntyre's (1984) concept of practice, the authors will advocate for virtue ethics as the essential component of professionalism and professional ethics in nursing. Finally, the case will be made for nursing to step forward and offer a transformational ethical framework to guide professional nursing education and practice.

A TIME OF DRAMATIC CHANGE

In the days following September 11, 2001, nursing programs all over the country experienced a surge of prospective students who decided that nursing was the career choice for them. Over and over, their words seemed to be the same: "I want to do something important; something that will make a [positive] difference. I want the opportunity to impact others' lives." These candidates' words were different from those who applied in the decades before. Often those prospective students said "I like science and I want to help people" when asked why they wanted a nursing career. After 9/11, applicants were speaking not just of the immediacy of results of their work but of a goal, or an ideal—a good—and came to their interviews conveying their willingness to work toward this meaningful goal.

These prospective students were describing their personal *teleological* orientation to nursing. The word *teleological* comes from the Greek word *telos* that means the end of a goal-directed process. Further, within the context of Greek traditional theory, this end or goal is considered something to which one should aspire—a good. Their aspirations anticipated a *change* in their lives as a result of this career choice. They envisioned nursing education as something beyond a transaction between teacher and student; they wanted and aspired to be part of a change. They were intentionally seeking a transformational experience.

FROM TRANSACTIONAL TO TRANSFORMATIONAL

Language has an important place in understanding human thought and action. It can be both a mirror and a light—sometimes language *reflects* change, and other times it *drives* change. From the 1960s until the end of the last century, nursing academic writing reflected one of two dominant, contemporary philosophical perspectives: social/historical constructivist paradigm that framed human activity as a social phenomenon, and the naturalistic paradigm or "things are as they are" view called *scientific realism* (Boyd, 2008). During this same period, healthcare ethics in the United States took a turn from community or collectivism and the common good to a strong focus on individual rights (Fan, 2006), leaving little room for virtue ethics and a contemplative view on how an individual might flourish in a healthcare environment. From the economic sector, business and global economics also grew in importance and the social contract became the fulcrum for all moral interactions (Cudd, 2009), reinforcing a social transactional goods and services and mutual agreement–oriented paradigm.

Nursing language has reflected these social and intellectual influences as the discipline has matured. Naturalistic, social transactional language is found in foundational American Nurses Association's (ANA) documents. The 1980 *Nursing: A Social Policy Statement* defines nursing as "the diagnosis and treatment of human responses to actual or potential health problems" (ANA, 1995, p. 6). The 2003 edition of ANA's *Nursing's Social Policy Statement* offers a broader, yet still largely transactional definition:

> Nursing is the protection, promotion, and optimization of health and abilities, prevention of illness and injury, alleviation of suffering through the diagnosis and treatment of human response, and advocacy in the care of individuals, families, communities, and populations. (p. 6)

Understandably the goal was to precisely describe what professional nurses do. In so doing, they also conveyed a contemporary transactional perspective for nursing.

A CHANGING WORLD VIEW: THE RETURN TO A
TRANSFORMATIONAL APPROACH

Beginning in the 1990s, powerful changes in healthcare organizations catalyzed a move from social and transactional language and thinking in nursing to a robust, transformational world view (Bleich & Kosiak, 2007) that clearly reflected ethical, prescriptive language. Words such as *best, good,* and *best practices* had not been part of the American academic nursing language, and were now being used. Clinical judgment no longer meant *using* clinical judgment, it meant using the *best* clinical judgment. *US News & World Report* began to identify the best hospitals ("America's Best Hospitals," 2009) and the best schools of nursing ("Rankings, Nursing," 2009); the National League for Nursing (NLN) began recognizing schools of nursing as Centers for Excellence (NLN, 2009). Although a part of today's language, the term *best* was largely absent from American nursing research literature just a decade ago. The word *best* appears seven times more frequently in the peer-reviewed research titles of the Cumulative Index to Nursing and Allied Health Literature (CINAHL) between 2000 and 2009 than during the 1990s. Even more dramatically, the term *best practice* appears in only eight peer reviewed research titles between 1990 and 2000, yet is 16 times more prevalent (128 titles) between 2000 and 2009.

Today, almost 6% of American healthcare organizations have achieved the American Nurses Credentialing Center's (ANCC) Magnet recognition status (ANCC, 2009b), with Magnet-like qualities such as autonomy, opportunity for professional advancement, and recognition are clearly identified in other studies of registered nurses' experiences (Buerhaus, Donelan, Ulrich, DesRoches, & Dittus, 2007). Based on quality indicators and standards of nursing practice, the ANCC's Magnet Recognition Program's attention to excellence exerts a sphere of influence that impacts health care nationally. Finally, the term *best practice* appears often in nursing literature, communicating evidence-based practices and appropriate standards of nursing care.

Transformational thinking is most evident in the scholarly work of leadership theory and practice. It successfully empowers people to reach beyond expectations by fostering a sense of ownership in achieving a larger vision (Grossman & Valiga, 2009). Because contemporary health care is a complex system of business and service, information access and the ensuing pressures of globalization pushed healthcare organizations to embrace transformative strategies with the hope of better managing structures, human resources, and the balance of profitability with quality (Bleich & Koziak, 2007). However, academic medicine and nursing by themselves did not have the tools to create such a change. Health care needed new knowledge from business, psychology, sociology, leadership, and economics to lead its transformation. Of particular interest was W. E. Deming's focus on quality management. His remarkable influence on the Japanese economy post–World War II (Simpson, 2009) offered a global model for transforming a workforce into one of high-quality and accompanying profit. Additionally, Deming advocated a strong program of education and self-improvement, with deliberate attention to the idea that pride of workmanship was necessary in order to achieve quality (Leadership Institute Inc., 2005). Porter-O'Grady and Malloch (2009), Grossman and Valiga, and others brought transformational leadership concepts to the nursing literature and into the national nursing spotlight. From the 1990s forward, a transformational approach to nursing practice and patient care quickly became an important part of the larger nursing conversation.

Now, nearly a decade since 9/11, the authors contend that a shift from a transactional mindset to a transformational worldview is one of the reasons that the American Nurses Credentialing Center (ANCC) Magnet Recognition Program has been so well received by practicing nurses; nurses understand the reason for Magnet goals because many of them entered nursing because of professional, self-described ideals that the Magnet Recognition Program can now help them meet.

The ANCC's Magnet Recognition Program models the success of this transformative perspective. Started in 1994, this program currently identifies 339 healthcare organizations as Magnet institutions (ANCC, 2009b). Fourteen forces of magnetism were identified as quality markers within nurses' work environments. The hope was that healthcare organizations possessing these qualities would attract and retain high-quality professionals and, in turn, provide excellent patient care (ANCC, 2009b). In 2008, the fourteen forces of magnetism were reclustered into five categories: transformational leadership, structural empowerment, exemplary professional practice, new knowledge, innovations and improvements, and empirical outcomes (ANCC, 2009c; Fig. 4-1).

Figure 4-1   New model for ANCC's Magnet Recognition Program.

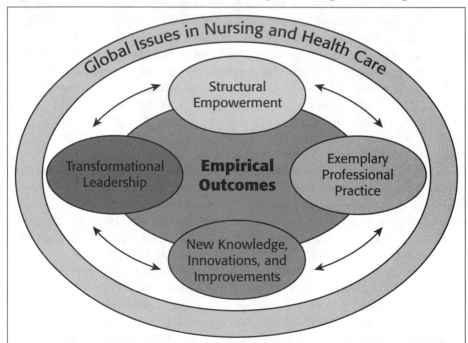

Table 4-1   Virtue Ethics Concepts Compared with ANCC's Magnet Recognition Program Goals

Concepts of virtue ethics (Hursthouse, 2009)	Goals of ANCC's Magnet Recognition Program
Excellence or virtue	Promoting quality in a setting that supports professional practice
Practical or moral wisdom	Identifying excellence in the delivery of nursing service to patients/residents
Happiness or flourishing	Disseminating best practices in nursing services

The ANCC's Magnet Recognition Program's goals are: (1) promoting quality in a setting that supports professional practice, (2) identifying excellence in the delivery of nursing service to patients/residents, and (3) disseminating best practices' in nursing services (ANCC, 2009a). Research findings indicate that implementing "Magnet hospital intervention was associated with a significantly improved nursing work environment as well as improved job-related outcomes for nurses and markers for quality of patient care" (Aiken, Buchan, Ball, & Rafferty, 2008, p. 3330) both in the United States and in the United Kingdom.

The impact of transformational language in nursing is much larger than a particular business model or strategic planning initiative. The word *transformational* compared with *transactional* points to a psychological component that goes beyond the idea of a social contract. Transformation assumes that there is change within the person and around the person, and that the change occurs over time. *Transformation also has ethical significance when normative language is used because transformation* assumes that the change can be assigned degrees of value such as *better* or *best*.

Virtue ethics ably explains the linguistic and operational transition within nursing during the past decade. Three concepts central to the ancient Greek traditions of virtue ethics (Hursthouse, 2009)—excellence or virtue (arête), practical or moral wisdom (phronesis), and happiness or flourishing (eudaimonia)—are implicit in the goals of the ANCC's Magnet Recognition Program (ANCC, 2009a; see Table 4-1). The ANCC's Magnet Recognition Program uses virtue ethics as its ethical foundation, bringing a new, strong theoretical basis to the change occurring in the discipline of nursing.

VIRTUE ETHICS AND THE FOUNDATIONS OF WESTERN THOUGHT

From the Greek perspective, all ethics are virtue ethics (MacIntyre, 1984) and, as such, human flourishing is a historically grounded foundational concept of Western thought and the human condition. Socrates proclaimed, ". . . it is not living which is of the most importance, but living well" (*Crito*, 49b, R. E. Allen translation). Aristotle began his most famous ethics treatise, *Nicomachean Ethics*, with the words, "Every art and every inquiry, and similarly every action and pursuit, is thought to aim at some good; and for this reason the good has rightly been declared to be that at which all things aim" (*Nicomachean Ethics*, I:1, Ross translation). Both Plato and Aristotle assert that character and values precede conduct and relationships. Values are embedded in what it is to know "the good," and are reflected in the character of the person (Godfrey, 1999). For the ancient Greeks, all knowledge is preexisting (*Posterior Analytics*, I:71, Revised Oxford translation); embedded within this knowledge is the notion of an ideal, or *telos*. This knowledge is not given to humans, but can be accessed through living a good life. By aiming for the good, one becomes a good person.

Assumptions of Virtue Ethics

These four assumptions are inherent in the study of virtue ethics:

1. An end, goal, or ideal (the "good," or *telos*) exists.
2. Humans are motivated to seek the good.
3. Virtues exist.
4. Virtues can be applied to seek and achieve a flourishing life.

An End, Goal, or Ideal (Telos) Exists

"[T]here is a *telos* which transcends the limited goods of practices by constituting the good of a whole human life" (MacIntyre, 1984, p. 203). Too often, those new to virtue ethics quickly dismiss the theory because perfection, of course, is not attainable. However, Aristotle did not argue for perfection. Instead, he said, "human good turns out to be activity of soul exhibiting excellence . . . in accordance with the best and most complete . . . life" (NE I:7). For Aristotle, the human good is the goal, the end, the ideal, and serves as a moral standard. He cautioned, however, that "we must add 'in a complete life.' For one swallow does not make a summer, and nor does one day; and so too one day, or a short time, does not make a man blessed and happy" (NE I:7). For Aristotle, it is very clear: "Every art and every inquiry, and similarly every action and pursuit, is thought to aim at some good" (NE I:1).

Humans Are Motivated to Seek the Good

As humans, we not only recognize that the good exists, but that we are also compelled to seek the good. "[T]he good has rightly been declared to be that at which all things aim" (NE I:1). Through seeking the good we will see the goods "that are attainable and achievable; for having this as sort of a pattern, we shall know better the goods that are good for us" (NE I:7). Said another way, seeking those goods that we can recognize as good helps us become aware of more goods that we might not ordinarily recognize. Therefore, seeking the good is morally equal to achieving the good. Using Aristotle's example of the shipbuilder seeking the good in building an excellent ship, a human being also seeks the overall good by aspiring to be a good human being (NE I:1).

Virtues Exist

Virtue is the state of character, which (1) makes one good and (2) makes the person perform his or her own work well (NE II:6). For Aristotle, virtue is neither a passion nor a faculty, but a state of being or a disposition, mediated and developed by experiences and choices. Further, "[v]irtue must have the quality of aiming at the intermediate" (NE II:6), and can be determined by practical wisdom.

Virtues Can Be Applied to Seek and Achieve a Flourishing Life

Aristotle defines the virtuous person as acting in accordance with the right rule, and that the framing of the rule is an intellectual operation (NE, Ross introduction, xv). He describes in more detail the states of mind necessary to reach the truth, but more importantly classifies these states of mind as requiring either intellectual resources (knowledge), or practice—or both. The most important message from this interchange (NE VI) is that virtue and, in turn, a flourishing life are achieved through habituation. One cannot know the right rule without intellectual work or practice or, in some cases, both. This means that no one person has more innate opportunity than another to the "good of a whole life" (MacIntyre, 1984, p. 203). The means for flourishing are open to all.

These four assumptions—that a goal that is good can be imagined, that it is a positive human quality to seek this goal, that virtues exist, and that through applying virtues one can achieve a flourishing life—form the foundation for Western thought about virtue ethics.

VIRTUE ETHICS AND THE FOUNDATIONS OF EASTERN THOUGHT

Fung Yu-lan, one of the great 20th-century authorities on historical Chinese thought, compares Confucius' influence in Chinese history with that of Socrates in the West. Confucius (551–479 BCE), according to Chinese tradition, was a thinker, political figure, and educator (Riegel, 2008). Fung Yu-lan taught about the education and comportment of the ideal man, using a "central Confucian understanding of virtue (*de*), which appreciates character cultivation and proper action as realized through exercising benevolence (*ren*) in the tasks of everyday life" (Fan, 2006, p. 546).

In Confucian thought, "virtue identifies a transformative power or moral energy that alters social relationships. It engages personal dynamism that relocates and properly orders the natural human inclinations and relationships" (Fan, 2006, p. 546). Combined actions to develop virtue and virtuous relationships result in one becoming morally worthy.

Confucianism is a dominant representation of Eastern philosophical and political thought, and is similar to the ancient Greek understanding of virtue ethics. First, the idea of an ideal man can be imagined and applied in making decisions about living a virtuous life. Second, virtue is a moral power that is exercised for the good of others and not for personal gain. Third, virtue is gained by habituation and teaching, not simply because humans have the capacity to understand what virtue means. Finally, the "transformative power or moral energy" (Fan, 2006, p. 546) of virtue communicates the dynamism that occurs when humans seek to live virtuously with the hope of having a fulfilling life. The East and the West have foundational similarities.

VIRTUE ETHICS AS CENTRAL TO A PRACTICE DISCIPLINE

Moving from the historical account of virtue ethic traditions into contemporary accounts, MacIntyre's (1984) work, *After Virtue*, is particularly helpful in explaining the relationship between *practice* and a specific, virtue-based moral philosophy. As MacIntyre says, "bricklaying is not a practice; architecture is. Planting turnips is not a practice; it is a skill. Farming is a practice" (p. 187). MacIntyre argues that a practice is much more than the completion of a series of tasks, no matter how complex. Using his definition, a practice always includes both *internal goods* and *standards of excellence*, and that by being part of a practice there is an inherent drive to strive for excellence. "[P]ractice is never just a set of technical skills, even when directed towards some unified purpose and even if the exercise of those skills can on occasion be valued or enjoyed for their own sake" (p. 193).

Further, MacIntyre (1984) claims a relationship that transcends the day-to-day practice environment. "To enter into a practice is to enter into a relationship not only with its contemporary practitioners, but also with those who have preceded us in the practice, particularly those whose achievements extended the reach of the practice to its present point" (p. 194). This conceptualization of practice and, by extension, the ability to teach practice to others, becomes a powerful way of explaining professionalism within any field of practice. One begins with individual transformation, develops a deeper understanding of the characteristics and responsibilities a practice can bring, moves closer toward the ideal of excellence, and then shares with others.

THE HISTORIAL CONTEXT: VIRTUE ETHICS IN NURSING

According to Hursthouse (2009), virtue ethics began with Plato and Aristotle and "persisted as the dominant approach in Western moral philosophy until at least the Enlightenment . . . with a momentary eclipse during the nineteenth century but re-emerged in the late 1950's in Anglo-American philosophy" (Hursthouse). Hursthouse's moral philosophy timeline differs significantly from what occurred in nursing, with virtue ethics' "momentary eclipse" occurring in the last half of the 20th century and just reemerging within the last decade or so. For the purposes of comparison, five eras of nursing history have been identified and are described:

- Period prior to professional nursing (Antiquity to 1579)
- Dark period of nursing (1580–1849)
- Nightingale period (1850–1910)
- Post-Nightingale period (1911–1955)
- Realism period (1956–1995)
- Teleological period (1996 to present)

Period Prior to Professional Nursing (Late Antiquity to 1579)

A number of colleagues (Dock & Stewart, 1938; Donahue, 1985; Smolan, Moffitt, & Naythons, 1990) describe the history of premodern nursing as the "the nursing impulse" (Donahue, 1985, p. 2). Donahue describes the time where nursing care most assuredly existed and was benevolently given (without formal education) without reward to oneself and usually through religious orders and societies. These religious institutions, particularly those within the Judeo-Christian tradition, communicated and reinforced the relational nature of nursing care, especially with vulnerable care recipients (Benner, 1997). The Christian values of equality and agape were clear in Christian teachings. St. Augustine's interest in neo-Platonic thought (*Confessions*, Pine-Coffin translation) strongly influenced his prolific early Roman Catholic Church writings. Equally, St. Thomas Aquinas's contributions to the theology of faith and reason were influenced by Aristotle. Aquinas's innovative theological ideas appeared at the beginning of the Renaissance, creating yet another way in which virtue ethics connected with the Western world centuries after it had first been introduced.

Dark Period of Nursing

Dock and Stewart (1938) refer to the dark period of nursing from 1580 to 1849, starting with the Protestant Reformation and the dissolution of Roman Catholic monasteries and convents, and ending with the advent of new thinking led by Florence Nightingale. According to Donahue (1985), the growing Protestant Church did not conceive its commitment to the sick and poor in the same central way that the Roman Catholic Church had. This led to poorer and poorer care, with little attention given to reform initiatives for all who fell ill.

A revolutionary change in political and philosophical thought occurred in the latter part of this period with the advent of the Age of Enlightenment (1688–1789). This period is often considered "the call for the independence of reason" (Sassen, 2008), when all previous assumptions of 18th-century European life were called into question. Although Enlightenment thinking in this period did not extend to social welfare reform, and therefore did not directly affect the care of the poor and sick, Florence Nightingale's extensive education in the classics and in Enlightenment writings left her well equipped to pioneer modern nursing in an age profoundly influenced by Enlightenment thinking. What nursing moral philosophy that could be found was still of the religious, benevolent nature of the earlier period.

Nightingale Period (1850–1910)

In the first half of the 19th century, nursing "was not work that could be seriously undertaken . . . by a young woman of good social standing. A hospital ward was considered to be no fit place for any modest woman of sound character and body" (Pavey, 1959, p. 276). Florence Nightingale (1820–1910) experienced a divine calling to become a nurse in 1837, yet because of her family's refusal to support her decision, was unable to take nurse's training until 1851. As her biographer Sir Edward Cook said, "she became a legend in her own lifetime" (Pavey, p. 273), beginning with her efforts in the Crimean War.

Nightingale's moral philosophy, and thus the moral philosophy for this 60-year period, is at once well-thought-through and complex, and difficult to discern. The author of nine books, Nightingale communicated both her firm understanding of nursing (i.e., *Notes on Nursing: What It Is and What It Is Not*) and her questions about theology and spirituality (*Suggestions for Thought: Selection and Commentaries*). There are, however, some aspects of her philosophical perspective that are evident through scholarly inquiry: She held an orientation to the general good (LeVasseur, 1998), possessed a transcendental world view (Porter, 2001), and considered the act of nursing to be an art requiring much preparation, with the body being medium for the art, "the temple of God's spirit" (Donahue, 1985, p. 469).

Post-Nightingale Period (1910–1955)

American schools of nursing were opened on the Nightingale plan in the 1870s and 1880s. "Miss Nightingale's uncompromising doctrine" (Dock & Stewart, 1938, p. 154) that the matron or the superintendent of the hospital be a nurse was not always adhered to in the United States, causing some controversy. The struggle between physicians and nurses was real, and would continue throughout the 20th century.

The post-Nightingale era in America seemed to be a time when nursing ideals and values were established, and reinforced. M. Adelaide Nutting (1926), nursing leader, wrote in 1926: "If nurses of the future work as loyally, as courageously, and as steadfastly, if they hold before them the vision of what nursing should be as faithfully as their sisters of the past have done, nursing will indeed come into her own" (p. 350). Nurses were valued, trained, and expected to perform in specific and self-sacrificing ways. Although this may not be an entirely positive viewpoint by today's standards, the virtue aspect of nursing in this period is clear.

Realism Period (1956–1995)

Fan (2006), in his work to develop a Confucian virtue bioethics, refers to the latter part of the 20th century as "a very particular era in American cultural heritage" (p. 542). He characterizes these changes as "(1) the deprofessionalization of American medicine which reduced it from a guild to a trade, (2) numerous movements on behalf of individual rights that in the United States that accented persons, especially patients, as individual, isolated decision-makers, and (3) the secularization of American society" (p. 542). Fan was speaking specifically of the bioethics movement, but the same forces were affecting nursing.

During this period, the Enlightenment ideals of individualism, reason, and critical questioning of all things traditional finally emerged within nursing. Schools of nursing discontinued capping and pinning ceremonies, hospital work attire changed from uniforms to scrubs, and traditional mores associated with nursing were questioned at all levels. At the same time, the profession developed into a discipline with research doctorates and a corresponding explosion of nursing knowledge.

Ethics in nursing underwent a drastic change, narrowing to address complicated ethical dilemmas seen in practice. Nursing followed the bioethics movement's lead and turned en mass to consequentialist and deontological theories for help in solving these problems. Autonomy, another term from the bioethics movement, became an important talking point in practice discussions. Finally, because virtue ethics (1) represented a traditional view of nursing and (2) was not in the current academic conversation, the topic was nearly absent from all reflective and research nursing literature in the United States (Godfrey, 1999).

Teleological Period (1996 to present)

Without question, health care and, in turn, nursing are strongly influenced by the transformational approach introduced by American business in the late 1990s and early 2000s. Whether or not the transformational and the explicit assumptions that accompany such language will develop into more than the business idea *du jour* and become part of larger thought in ethics in American nursing remains to be seen.

Several factors may catalyze such a move. First, the 50-year period when normative language (including the *good* and the *good nurse*) disappeared from American nursing discourse did not occur in other countries (Godfrey, 1999). Nursing thinkers across the globe have continued to conceptualize nursing in ways that include all three dominant moral philosophy perspectives: deontology, consequentialism, and virtue ethics. Advancing an empirical view of nursing science may not include substantive research efforts in virtue ethics; however, advancing professionalism within the discipline likely will.

Second, the evidence-based practice movement that began in England is defined in distinctively normative, superlative language. Evidence-based practice is the "conscientious, explicit and judicious use of current best evidence in making decisions about individual patients" (Sackett, Rosenberg, Gray, Haynes, & Richardson, 1996). Because American medicine and nursing have so heartily embraced the evidence-based practice initiative, it may be that normative language will become more accepted. Finally, other disciplines have taken a serious look at virtue ethics as a significant method to describe and develop their body of knowledge and practice (Fine & Teram, 2009; Sox, 2007; Sullivan, 2005; Sylvester, 2002). Influence from other fields can and should be a force for change in both academics and practice, enhancing nursing rather than smothering its distinctiveness as a profession.

Will American nursing engage in the conversation to develop a more comprehensive and integrative view of professionalism and professional ethics for nursing? And will professionalism be viewed as a primarily ethical endeavor, that incorporates the idea of *telos*—a concept that, except for a 50-year hiatus in the United States, has been an integral part of both ancient and modern nursing—throughout the world?

REFERENCES

Aiken, L. H., Buchan, J., Ball, J., & Rafferty, A. M. (2008). Transformative impact of Magnet designation: England case study. *Journal of Clinical Nursing, 17*(24), 3330–3337.

America's best hospitals. (2009). *US News & World Report*. Available at: http://health.usnews .com/health/best-hospitals. Accessed July 30, 2009.

American Nurses Association. (1995). *Nursing's social policy statement*. Washington, DC: Author.

American Nurses Association. (2003). *Nursing's social policy statement* (2nd ed.). Washington, DC: Author.

American Nurses Credentialing Center. (2009a). *Goals of the program*. Available at: http:// www.nursecredentialing.org/Magnet/ProgramOverview/GoalsoftheMagnetProgram.aspx. Accessed July 30, 2009.

American Nurses Credentialing Center. (2009b). *Growth*. Available at: http://www .nursecredentialing.org/Magnet/ProgramOverview/GrowthoftheProgram.aspx. Accessed July 30, 2009.

American Nurses Credentialing Center. (2009c). *New model*. Available at: http://www .nursecredentialing.org/Magnet/ResourceCenters.aspx. Accessed July 30, 2009.

Benner, P. (1997). A dialogue between care ethics and virtue ethics. *Theoretical Medicine, 18*(1–2), 47–61.

Bleich, M. R., & Kosiak, C. P. (2007). Managing, leading and following. In P. Yoder-Wise (Ed.), *Leading and managing in nursing* (4th ed., pp. 3–25). St. Louis, MO: Mosby.

Boyd, R. (2008). Scientific realism. In E. N. Zalta (Ed.), *The Stanford encyclopedia of philosophy*. Available at: http://plato.stanford.edu/archives/fall2008/entries/scientific-realism/. Retrieved August 2, 2009.

Buerhaus, P. I., Donelan, K., Ulrich, B. T., DesRoches, C., & Dittus, R. (2007). Trends in the experiences of hospital-employed registered nurses: Results from three national surveys. *Nursing Economics, 25*(2), 69–80.

Cudd, A. (2009). Contractarianism. In E. N. Zalta (Ed.), *The Stanford encyclopedia of philosophy*. Available at: http://plato.stanford.edu/archives/fall2008/entries/contractarianism/. Retrieved August 2, 2009.

Dock, L. L., & Stewart, I. M. (1938). *A short history of nursing: From earliest times to the present day*. New York: G. P. Putnam's Sons.

Donahue, M. P. (1985). *Nursing: The finest art*. St. Louis, MO: C. V. Mosby.

Fan, R. (2006). Towards a Confucian virtue bioethics: Reframing Chinese medical ethics in a market economy. *Theoretical Medicine and Bioethics, 27,* 541–566.

Fine, M., & Teram, E. (2009). Believers and skeptics: Where social worker situate themselves regarding the Code of Ethics. *Ethics and Behavior, 19*(1), 60–78.

Fung, Y. (1948). Some prominent characteristics of historical Chinese thought. In *A short history of Chinese philosophy*. New York: Macmillan.

Godfrey, N. (1999). *Character and ethical behavior of nurses*. Dissertation. University of Missouri-Columbia.

Grossman, S. C., & Valiga, T. M. (2009). *The new leadership challenge* (3rd ed.). Philadelphia: F. A. Davis Co.

Hursthouse, R. (2009). Virtue ethics. In E. N. Zalta (Ed.), *The Stanford encyclopedia of philosophy*. Available at: http://plato.stanford.edu/archives/spr2009/entries/ethics-virtue/.

Leadership Institute Inc. (2005). *Who is Dr. W. Edwards Deming?* Available at: http://www.lii.net /deming.html. Accessed July 30, 2009.

LeVasseur, J. (1998). Student scholarship, Plato, Nightingale, and contemporary nursing. *Image: Journal of Nursing Scholarship, 30*(3), 281–285.

MacIntyre, A. (1984). *After virtue* (2nd ed.). Notre Dame, IN: University of Notre Dame Press.

National League for Nursing. (2009). *Centers of excellence*. Available at: http://www.nln .org/excellence/coe/index.htm. Accessed July 30, 2009.

Nutting, M. E. (1926). *A sounder economic basis for schools of nursing*. New York: Putnam.

Pavey, A. E. (1959). *The story of the growth in nursing as an art, a vocation and a profession*. London: Faber & Faber Ltd.

Porter-O'Grady, T., & Malloch, K. (2009). Leaders of innovation: Transforming postindustrial healthcare. *Journal of Nursing Administration, 39*(6), 245–248.

Porter, S. (2001). Nightingale's realist philosophy of science. *Nursing Philosophy, 2*(1), 14–25.

Rankings, nursing. (2009). *US News & World Report*. Available at: http://grad-schools.usnews .rankingsandreviews.com/best-graduate-schools/top-nursing-schools/rankings. Accessed July 30, 2009.

Riegel, J. (2008). Confucius. In E. N. Zalta (Ed.), *The Stanford encyclopedia of philosophy*. Available at: http://plato.stanford.edu/archives/fall2008/entries/confucius. Accessed August 2, 2009.

Sackett, D. L., Rosenberg, W. M., Gray, J. A., Haynes, R. B., & Richardson, W. S. (1996). Evidence based medicine: What it is and what it isn't. *British Medical Journal, 13*(312), 71–72.

Sassen, B. (2008). 18th century German philosophy prior to Kant. In E. N. Zalta (Ed.), *The Stanford encyclopedia of philosophy*. Available at: http://plato.stanford.edu/archives/fall2008 /entries/18thGerman-preKant/. Accessed August 2, 2009.

Simpson, R. I. (2009). Innovations in transforming organizations. *Nursing Administration Quarterly, 33*(3), 268–272.

Smolan, R., Moffitt, P., & Naythons, M. (1990). *The power to heal: Ancient arts and modern medicine.* New York: RxMedia Group.

Sox, H. C. (2007). The ethical foundations of professionalism: A sociologic history. *Chest, 131,* 1532–1540.

Sullivan, W. M. (2005). *Work and integrity: The crisis and promise of professionalism in America* (2nd ed.). San Francisco: Jossey-Bass.

Sylvester, C. (2002). Ethics and the quest for professionalization. *Therapeutic Recreation Journal, 36*(4), 314–334.

CHAPTER 5

A Framework for Nurse Professionals

All natural goods perish.
Can things whose end is always dust
and disappointment be the real good
which our souls require?

—WILLIAM JAMES, 1902

A recentering of professionalism as both psychological and social, and an inclusion of a method for character development through virtue ethics, are evident in the literature of professionalism and professional ethics. For the individual within the context of professional practice, ethics broadens into a transformational rather than transactional experience.

As our work on this book progressed, we discovered and became firmly convinced that a nurse professional's work, both decisions and actions, are strongly ethical in nature. Professional ethics and ethics in general are so enmeshed with the conceptualization of professionalism that it is difficult to separate the two. Nursing practice occurs through a series of decisions; almost every decision and action of a nurse professional has ethical import. Separating professionalism from ethics is like separating parts of the body. The eyes are separate from the heart, or the brain from the big toe, but each is necessary and they function as a whole.

However, the study of professionalism does not stop with professionalism, ethics, and our metaphor of body parts. Other disciplines, like psychology and the study of moral development, philosophy, history, cognitive study of the mind, sociology, religion, business, law, and the applied disciplines like physical therapy, medicine, dentistry, and nursing contribute to our understanding of professionalism. The proposed framework, the Framework for Nurse Professionals (FrNP), is a synthesis, or unity, of ideas. As authors, we have taken the liberty of simplifying, organizing, and conceptualizing bits and pieces from many sources. There are often watershed phenomena that occur in the literature, where a number of authors come to similar conclusions. Work in professionalism is one of those instances and, as such, there is little originality. This conceptualization is what has been gleaned through others.

The primary focus of this chapter is to introduce the FrNP and the accompanying Stairstep Model of Professional Transformation (Stairstep model) to more fully convey the richness of professionalism and professional ethics to those aspiring to become nurse professionals. A final section describes how the FrNP is particularly helpful in addressing (1) fragmentation, (2) wrongdoing within the profession, and (3) justification of the use of narrative.

A TRANSFORMATIONAL, ETHICAL FRAMEWORK FOR NURSE PROFESSIONALS (FrNP)

Concepts of the Framework

To begin the explanation of the FrNP, the reader is directed to Figure 5-1. The three main sections of the figure correspond to the three main moral components of FrNP: the *moral agent* and the elements that the agent considers in determining how to live as a professional; *phronesis* or the process of deliberation, making fitting choices, and acting on those choices; and the *outcome*, or *telos*, that impacts both the moral agent and the practice in which the agent is engaged. The FrNP represents the dynamic interplay of these elements as a life process that occurs over time.

The Moral Agent

The moral agent in the FrNP is the nurse professional or student making the transition to living the life of the nurse professional. The moral agent brings

Figure 5-1   Framework for nurse professionals: The transformational process.

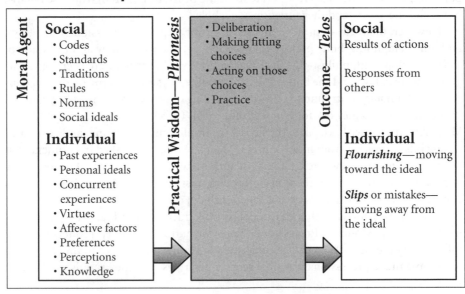

the *social* and *psychological* dimensions of self to any instance where the need to think/say/act (applying phronesis, or practical wisdom) is necessary. The *social* dimension of the agent corresponds to the deontological tradition of duties, principles, and rights that are primarily transactional in nature, and communicate how we relate to others. The nurse brings multiple social elements such as cultural norms, laws, rules, faith-based expectations, and perceptions of the social ideal and the ideal self as the nurse perceives others see him or her. From a sociological professional perspective, the nurse professional attempts to conform to what society and the profession expects. These include the practice acts as designated by the government, as well as standards, mores, and ethical codes of professional organizations. This combination of expectations together combine the social professional ideal.

The *psychological* dimension of self and the *ideal self* are linked closely to identity and are the nurse's expectations of him or herself—who one believes one "should" be. Other psychological elements come into play and influence the ideal self and reflect the totality of what makes up the internal world of the individual. Internal elements can include past life and professional experiences, virtues, a sense of balance, methods for making decisions and habituated skills, knowledge, a *personal professional ideal* of what the nurse expects of himself or herself in particular situations or contexts, developmental levels, personal faith, communication skills, and critical thinking skills, just to name a portion of what comprises the inner world.

Virtues have a prominent place in the FrNP and are broadly defined as traits or characteristics of a good person that enables him or her to work well (Pellegrino & Thomasma, 1993, p. 5). Virtues, as Aristotle described, approximate what is now known in contemporary psychology as states and traits. For the purpose of the FrNP virtues can be either *trait* or *state*. A virtue *trait* is a more stable quality of character; an individual has a trait or proclivity to make choices and act in certain ways *naturally*—but this is not a virtue. The natural proclivity becomes a virtue of excellence when one knows that there is a choice and applies the virtue to the situation for the right reason and in the right way. Virtues guide the moral agent toward the *telos*, being a person of excellence who practices a profession well.

The virtue *state* is more fluid and changeable. *State* is how the virtue is manifested in given situations. As stated previously, the development of the virtue trait or character occurs with multiple proper application of the virtue state to given situations.

In instances in which a virtue is not fully manifested in the right way, we borrow from the mistakes literature and use the word *slip* (Leape, 2000). A slip occurs when one does not use a virtue properly, and good outcomes are compromised. Although Leape used the term to refer to action only, in the FrNP it can refer to wrong thinking as well as wrong doing.

Phronesis: Using Virtues Well

Phronesis is also referred to as practical wisdom and is the *ability* of the agent to use virtues appropriately in given situations. Phronesis includes both thinking by using virtues well in making decisions and in following through with actions decisions made. Using the virtues well also improves one's ability to learn and sharpen moral sensitivity and response. Pellegrino and Thomasma (1993) identified good use of virtue as the ability to "strike a balance between two extremes," the emotional and the cognitive and to "unify the person toward an end" or the *telos* (p. 28).

Outcome: Flourishing

In a general sense, the term *outcome* means that the facts are in and the evaluation is imminent. The FrNP expands the notion of evaluation from a purely descriptive "what is" approach, to also include a normative component, asking the question, "what should be?" or "how should we have acted?" It is this normative perspective that affirms that a personal ideal of what a professional should be exists and can be sought, and that one can make decisions and act in ways that move the individual closer to achieving or further away the ideal, depending on one's choices. When virtues are used appropriately through phronesis or practical wisdom and unify one toward the *telos*, the natural aspiration of the individual nurse is to be a person and professional of excellence and to do good work.

One final element of the ancient Greek virtue ethics tradition remains to be introduced: that of eudaimonia, translated as *flourishing, happiness*, or *living the good life* and is what comes from an awareness of *telos* and the positive impact that one receives in striving to reach it. This sense of flourishing, gained through recognition that an ideal exists and that something good is gained by striving to attain that ideal, is a result that is potentially far more meaningful to a nurse professional than a transactional, descriptive assessment of one's actions. Striving toward an ideal, or *telos*, leads to a sense of flourishing and, as such, enables the professional to more clearly articulate what it means to be a professional who is responding to a calling and serving the needs of society.

The limited virtue ethics research in nursing supports the notion that nurses already possess a virtue orientation (Robertson, 1996; Smith & Godfrey, 2002), and it develops as a result of nursing practice itself—the doing and being of nursing. Just as flourishing occurs through the process of striving toward the *telos*, so nursing practice occurs through the everyday activities of the professional that in turn are nursing practice (Pellegrino & Thomasma, 1993). Aristotle used the example of building a ship. The builders work toward completion of a seaworthy vessel, their practice is to complete the building of ships, but the *telos* aims at the best ship that can be and the good that comes from it.

When considering the difference between work and practice, work constitutes the actions that, when taken that together, accomplish good practice. The checking of vital signs, the comforting and communicating with a patient, and identifying patient problems are work toward the goal or end of good nursing practice. Pellegrino and Thomasma (1993) advocated that the end/goal for the practice of medicine be the healing relationship and that this conception be added to the traditional four principles of nonmaleficence, beneficence, autonomy, and justice. Although much could be said about the end and practice of nursing, simply stated, for our purposes, practice is work done by the nurse professional that achieves good through a therapeutic relationship that is empowering the recipients of nursing care, reducing suffering, improving health, and, when appropriate, facilitating a good death. The practice of nursing in turn shapes the nurse as he or she lives life as a nurse professional.

For example, Nurse G is striving toward passing her NCLEX. As she prepares she flourishes, envisioning passing the test as part of her personal professional ideal (and clearly the socially constructed professional ideal). She is being transformed through the process. The *telos*, the ideal of the good is motivating her to *be the best she can be. Here is the ideal set before you, strive for it,* she tells herself. It becomes part of the accomplishments that move her toward becoming the ideal nurse.

The ideal is futuristic because one never truly accomplishes the personal professional ideal completely. Once Nurse G passed her examination, she perceives herself as closer to the ideals of a nurse professional, but this accomplishment does not mean that she has finished and is now deemed to be a nurse professional. Rather, she continues to strive for further development and achievement of her ideal, which also unfolds over time. At same time she sees the benefit in her work. Nurse G is becoming a good nurse who does good work. She is engaged in a process of living a professional life.

THE STAIRSTEP MODEL OF PROFESSIONAL TRANSFORMATION

The FrNP is designed to communicate a unified model of deontology, consequentialism, and virtue ethics within a nursing context, showing movement and progress as the nurse grows as a nurse professional, all the while recognizing that no one is perfect and that the ideal can never truly be achieved. While useful in a foundational way and essential as a beginning point in further scholarly theory development and empirical research, the authors believed that a second, simple representation is needed to help nursing students and those already in practice to have a clearer vision of their own transformational journey. For simplification purposes, the Stairstep Model of Professional Transformation (Stairstep model;

see Fig. 5-2) was developed. Three central ideas are communicated: (1) the place of principle-based ethics, consequentialist ethics, and virtue ethics in professional transformation; (2) the dynamic nature of flourishing and of making mistakes (slips); and (3) how a larger view of professional formation and transformation can help nursing students and nurses embrace a broader understanding of the discipline that is commensurate with the recognition and trust that nursing receives from society as a whole.

Figure 5-2   The Stairstep Model of Professional Transformation.

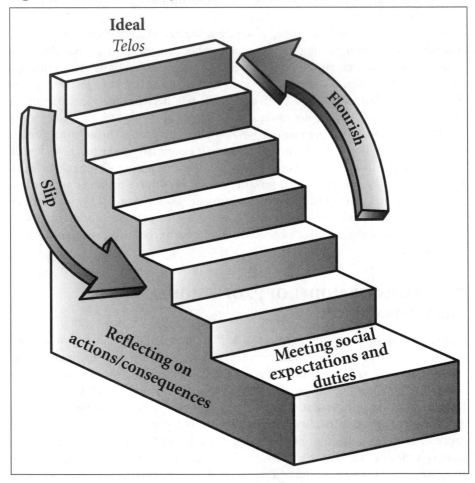

Deontology, Consequentialism, and Virtue

Deontological, or principle-based ethics, focuses on the intent of the agents and the subsequent recognition of duties communicated through codes, standards, and social professional expectations. The licensing process, regulatory actions by state boards of professional nursing, and the code of ethics for nurses (American Nurses Association, 2001) are examples of social professional expectations and are represented lower on the staircase, affirming that these codes and standards are known social expectations from the beginning of one's nursing practice.

Consequentialist ethical thought, in its purest form, weighs the value of any decision based on the outcome of greatest good for the greatest number. Although this thinking is a critical element in most dilemma ethics exercises, it has less of a place in everyday ethics when professional transformation is a consistent goal. However, reflection on one's actions and their consequences can be important in professional development, and does inform the professional about the norms of others and the discipline in general. Therefore, reflecting on actions and their consequences appears at the base of the staircase—used as a part of one's professional development to foster growth and understanding.

From a virtue perspective, the motivation and outcomes are dependent on the agent making virtues work well so that good choices and practices result. The personal life and the professional life of the moral agent represent a series of events over time and are likened to climbing a staircase. The top tier of the staircase, the good to which one aspires, represents the *telos*, or the ideal. This ideal is a combination of the socially constructed professional ideal and the personal professional ideal.

The Dynamic Nature of Flourishing and of Making Mistakes

Just as the process of striving for *telos* produces flourishing and transformation of the nurse professional, good work further reinforces the proper use of virtues that, in turn, reinforces character development. Nurse professionals then perceive themselves as flourishing and closer to realizing personally, professionally, and socially constructed ideals. If a nurse professional uses phronesis well and makes balanced decisions, he or she hopefully contributes to the personal/professional good, bring about good work, and move closer to the ideal—and, figuratively, take a step up the staircase.

However, if the stair climbing nurse professional descends rather than ascends the stair steps, he or she has made a slip. A slip is the condition in which an individual has used the virtues or other agent specific elements less fitting and in ways that do not conform to the agent's ethical ideal—either the internal personal/professional ideal and/or to the external socially constructed ideal.

A Larger View of Professional Transformation

How does this new conceptualization of professionalism benefit nursing education and nursing practice? In addition to offering a broader and applied view of ethical traditions, the FrNP and the Stairstep model teaching tools address personal professional development and conceptualize professionalism as a lifelong dynamic process that is goal directed. Such an approach gives voice to nurses who before have not found adequate words to express their own sense of meaning and professional growth gained through their work. Students just entering the intellectual study of nursing will have additional language to convey why the study is so hard and the learning can be exhausting. Finally, a heightened sense of professional awareness and transformation may help some nurses see their work and their calling with renewed encouragement. Seeing one's chosen profession as an open field of possibilities is far better than thinking only of the regulatory constraints, costs of licenses and continuing education, and mandatory inservices in the workplace.

THORNY ISSUES

Three thorny problems—wrongdoing in the profession, fragmentation of the self, and the need for narrative and reflexivity—were raised at earlier points in the text. The FrNP and the corresponding Stairstep model is helpful in more fully explaining these issues. The FrNP suggests practical approaches to handle them in nursing education and practice.

Wrongdoing in the Profession

There is no complete explanation for making mistakes or slips in clinical practice without considering nurses as individual moral agents rather than as social aggregates. Errors in clinical practice, theory development, and methods to avoid and deal with mistakes have been a topic of great interest in the healthcare field.

Martin (1999) labeled errors and mistakes more broadly as wrongdoing among professionals. Wrongdoing results from either intentional or unintentional decisions and actions. Errors and mistakes are wrongdoing that is unintentional in nature. The individual agent does not intend a negative outcome. Mistakes occur from *psychological* causes of either insufficient knowledge or from character issues such as lack of attentiveness, weakness, absence of proper use of virtues, or egoism. Egoism, in a professional setting, is a response that places the individual moral agent's benefit before that of the patient or recipient of care.

Sociological influences from outside an individual moral agent may also contribute to wrongdoing or mistakes. The external influence includes people, groups, institutions, or governments. Internal and external worlds create a tension between what the person believes they should do and social expectations. If the internal and external worlds are incommensurable, the individual sacrifices either his or her personal professional ideal of who he or she expects himself or herself to be and do as a moral agent or his or her perceived social ideal and of the expectations of specific institutions or professional groups. In either case, moral distress may result.

Let us turn to the case of Nurse T, a newly graduated nurse professional. The culture on the nursing unit where she works is resistant to flourishing. The nursing staff members have little motivation to improve themselves professionally or to improve care. Nurses provide standard care and spend 1 to 2 hours at the end of the shift doing paperwork and talking. Nurse T recognizes the expectation of the unit, but would rather chart over the course of the shift and spend time with patients at the end of the shift. Nurse T feels badly. The other staff view her as idealistic and inexperienced. She has not developed the virtue of bravery well enough to break the expected routine and respond to her personal professional ideal rather than the social expectations of the pathological culture on the unit. If asked, Nurse T would say she is "just chicken." She knows what she should do but does not carry it out. She has thought about finding other life work and that perhaps nursing just is not right for her.

In this case, Nurse T is responding in an egoistic way, to conform, and placing her own interests above that of patients' interests. At the same time, she senses shame and moral distress because she is not acting bravely. If Nurse T were to act in a nonconforming way and provide better care, she would use the virtue of bravery well and provide better care for her patients.

Wrongdoing in professional practice can occur as a purely psychological or a sociological influence, but most often results from a combination of both. Mistakes are thought to be a multiplicity of precarious elements coming together that create a perfect storm (Crigger, 2005). Without involving the individual moral agent there is no full account of mistakes, wrongdoing, or egoism. In the Stairstep model (Fig. 5-2) mistakes are evident as "slips," with an arrow pointing downward to indicate regression on the stairway.

Fragmentation of the Self

Another significant problem that results from the use of the exclusive use of a socially constructed professional is the fragmentation, compartmentalization, and loss of integrity of the self. The fragmented self lacks good use of the virtue integrity. 'Integrity' originated from Latin and means wholeness or completeness. The word describes an ability of the self, or individual, to be consistent in relationship with everyone and everything in the world. Integrity will be further discussed in Chapter 8, but is described here because of its importance in understanding fragmentation and compartmentalization of the professional and personal life.

The psychological self is essential for creating a sense of personal and professional wholeness. The ability of the moral agent doing the right thing even if no one is looking demonstrates personal commitment to the good use of integrity. The nurse of integrity reports an error made in giving a medication, completes a treatment administration under difficult circumstances, and charts only the clinical findings that were really observed and tested.

The person who lacks integrity and who lives life only as a series of social roles is at risk of becoming fragmented. A fragmented self means that there is no individual character to offer consistency and glue together the different social roles that one assumes. The individual person is but a uniform with no one inside, or a hook, as suggested by MacIntyre (1981), on which social roles are hung. No more dramatic compartmentalization of social roles and fragmentation exists than that of the fictitious Dr. Jekyll and Mr. Hyde. Mr. Hyde was cruel and motivated by base instincts while Dr. Jekyll appeared a mild mannered man who practiced his profession well. Like the story, the fragmented individual is one who is able to reconcile professional roles with personal ones even though there may be inconsistencies.

Nurse W is stellar at her work, but has a double life. She is abusive to her children and is unfaithful to her husband. Can Nurse W maintain the disparate roles: one as an excellent professional and the other as an unethical wife and mother? Her personal integrity is lacking and she is unable to realistically view the disparity. The sociological paradigm would suggest that she can partition and play each role seperately, while a character based ethic suggests that she cannot. Like Jekyll and Hyde, there is a potential risk for the corrupted self to bleed into the good professional or for those outside of the self to view the disparity and condemn it.

Narrative and Reflection

Reflection and the use of narrative in nursing education has always been part of our educational strategy. Both rest on an assumption of the personal psychological self. There must be a psychological self who is able to self-evaluate. William James, who has been called the father of American psychology, saw the absurdity of omission of self psychology. "No psychology," James wrote, "can question the *existence* of personal selves" (1890/1950, p. 226).

Knowledge- and content-based education can crowd out the time for reflective thinking. With use of the FrNP and virtue ethics tradition, focus of the self, including self-discovery and self-evaluation, is essential. Professional nursing education is brought to life with greater reflection and personal stories about practice and through development of the ideal—as one author called it, the "ethical self portrait" (Harris, 2008).

Benner, Tanner, and Chesla (2009) highly recommend the use of narrative as a transformational strategy for nursing, and other disciplinary conversations reflect the same enthusiasm. Developing as an integrated, mature moral agent is closely tied to self-reflection and the use of a narrative ethic.

With a union of the psychological and social paradigms, the rich inner world of the individual adds a vibrant dimension. So much of what we see in ethics in nursing that animates our ethical senses comes from exploration of the inner world and of lived experiences. Besides being a philosopher and psychologist, William James was also well known for his metaphors. One of particular relevance was James' comparison of a menu to the real meal. The restaurant menu, or as James called it, the bill of fare, may tell you what you will eat but, as informative as a menu might be, it is not the real meal—the steak and fries. Printed words have little more in common with the smell and taste of real food than to transmit knowledge of what can be obtained for a meal if the cook delivers. In this case, without the real meal, without contextualization of the inner world and the nexus of relationships with others, professionalism is like the menu and not the meal itself.

The poverty of traditional ethics has stimulated a greater respect for subjectivity and contextualization through caring theory and narrative ethics. Narrative ethics and literary theory are often combined, elevating individual narratives to a central role in teaching and understanding ethics. In fact, use of narratives plays a significant role in bioethics (Nelson, 1997) but may often turn toward the objective and detachedment from the ethical situation rather than engaging in a "real meal." Nussbaum (1987) vividly described her encounter of understanding the difference between thinking about ethics and engaging in ethical life. After reading Derrida and using Nietszche's metaphor, Nussbaum (1987) claimed, "I feel a certain hunger for blood—that is, for writing about literature that talks of human lives and choices as if they matter to us all" (p. 58).

Whether blood or steak and fries, that which has meaning reflects the sameness of everyday living as well as the passion of human suffering and can only be fully realized by real people who make real choices and have real experiences as they live real lives. Narrative ethics, whether case study, literature, or other art forms, is and will continue to be a methodology that will keep ethics, professional ethics, and professionalism real.

BENEFITS OF THE FRNP AND THE STAIRSTEP MODEL

The visual conceptualizations offered in Figures 5-1 and 5-2 offer a comprehensive view of professionalism that can be encouraging to students entering the discipline and practicing nurses for whom meaning has diminished. Moral agency is fully addressed, making room for both psychological and sociological perspectives. Further, the framework establishes justification for teaching character development in professionalism as an explicit part of the curriculum. Professional development is both aspirational with a striving toward the ideal self and *telos* and transformational as the process of striving toward the desired ends unfolds.

The FrNP explains and offers ways to address some of the problems that have plagued professionalism, ethics, and professional ethics when less comprehensive conceptions are used. One of the most refreshing and bold ideas that emerges from this framework is that of hope for change. As a professional living a process over time, one can view professionalism as a way of growing that is accomplished through acceptance of slips as an anticipated part of growth, rather than as a source of shame, moral distress, and condemnation. Slips are no longer exceptions that occur from a bad, lazy, or dumb nurse, but rather become part of a way in which nurse professionals flourish.

REFERENCES

American Nurses Association. (2001). *Code of ethics for nurses*. Washington, DC: Author.

Benner, P., Tanner, C. A., & Chesla, C. A. (2009). *Expertise in nursing* (2nd ed.). New York: Springer Publishing Company.

Crigger, N. (2005). Two models of mistake-making in professional practice: Moving out of the closet. *Nursing Philosophy, 6*, 11–18.

Harris, C. E. (2008). The good engineer: Giving virtue its due in engineering ethics. *Science Engineering Ethics, 14*(2), 153–164.

James, W. (1890/1950). *The principles of psychology*. New York: Dover.

Leape, L. L. (2000). Error in medicine. In S. B. Rubin & L. Zoloth (Eds.), *Margin of error* (pp. 95–111). Hagerstown, MD: University Publishing Group.

MacIntyre, A. (1981). *After virtue: A study in moral theory*. Notre Dame, IN: University of Notre Dame Press.

Martin, M. (1999). Explaining wrongdoing in professions. *Journal of Social Philosophy, 30*(2), 236–250.

Nelson, H. L. (1997). Introduction: How to do things with stories. In H. L. Nelson (Ed.), *Stories and their limits narrative approaches to bioethics* (pp. vii–xx). New York: Routledge.

Nussbaum, M. C. (1987). Perceptive equilibrium: literary theory and ethical theory. *LOGOS: Philosophical Issues in Christian Perspective, 8*, 516–529.

Pellegrino, E. D., & Thomasma, D. C. (1993). *The virtues in medical practice*. New York: Oxford University Press.

Robertson, D. W. (1996). Ethical theory, ethnography, and differences between doctors and nurses in approaches to patient care. *Journal of Medical Ethics, 22*, 292–299.

Smith, K. V., & Godfrey, N. S. (2002). Being a good nurse and doing the right thing: A qualitative study. *Nursing Ethics, 9*(3), 301–312.

SECTION 3

How Can Professionalism Be Taught?

CHAPTER 6

Learning a Profession:
Considerations and Strategies

More than any other type of occupation,
professions are critically determined
by the education of their members.

—SULLIVAN, COLBY, WEGNER, BOND,
AND SHULMAN, 2007

The overarching purpose, or *telos*, for nurse professionals is to be good nurses who do good work. However, the conception of what "good" is has long been criticized as relativistic and vague. Aristotle acknowledged that good is, in its final consideration, decided on by individuals. Though individual perceptions of the good are important, society also addresses the good. The nursing profession and each nurse professional appears to be closer to consensus about at least some aspects of what is good work. There is substantial evidence that nursing practice is informing and, likewise, is informed by professionalism and ethical theory. Understanding of the good is emergent in how nurses employ the notion of the good in everyday practice (Benner, Sutphen, Leonard-Kahn, & Day, 2008; O'Connor, 2007; Smith & Godfrey, 2002), yet, despite the current work toward a clearer articulation of professionalism, it is likely that understanding of the good and its contribution to professionalism and ethics may remain part of the informal or hidden curriculum expressed largely through student–faculty interaction (Billings & Halstead, 2009). If a change toward a more explicit and transformational conceptualization of professionalism is anything like research dissemination, it may take nurse educators years to adopt a radically different approach to professional education.

Nurse educators will themselves need to understand the complex business of teaching professionalism theory and formation in order to facilitate students' learning in undergraduate and graduate curricula. In this chapter, the authors first examine ways in which other disciplines have addressed professional education. Next, a synthesis of the emergent trends seen in other disciplines and nursing is discussed, and, last, we offer recommendations for a well-grounded professionalism initiative in nursing education.

EDUCATION WITHIN THE PROFESSIONS

Renewed interest in professionalism has transformed education in many professions. A landmark interdisciplinary study entitled Preparation for the Professions, by the

Carnegie Foundation for Advancement of Teaching identified three high-end apprenticeships: the cognitive apprenticeship, the skill-based or hands-on apprenticeship, and the apprenticeship that fosters ethical comportment (Benner, Tanner, & Chesla, 2009). Five professions were studied—ministry, law, engineering, nursing, and medicine—using these three dimensions of or apprenticeships for professional education (The Carnegie Foundation for the Advancement of Teaching, 2009c). A brief discussion of the findings for each of the five disciplines is presented.

Ministry

Foster, Dahill, Golemon, and Tolentino (2006) found that ministry clustered its professional preparation into "a cognitive or intellectual apprenticeship, a practical apprenticeship of skill, and an apprenticeship of identity formation" (p. 5). Traditional academic settings—classrooms, exams, reading, lectures—have a place, but the classroom is only part of the reality of professional education for ministers. In ministry, there is a need to be "directly concerned with how to *be* in the world" (p. 6). Foster et al. (2006) use the term *symbolic analysis* to explain traditional academic work, confirming that much of what is learned in ministry takes place outside the classroom environment and is relational in nature and focused for the recipients of ministerial care.

Yale Divinity School's reflective-practitioner approach is an example of how to *be* in the world and how to engage the students' moral formation within a formalized academic setting (Foster et al., 2006). Dr. Barbara Blodgett prepared students for internships at Yale Divinity School and uses reflection-in-action based on Schon's (1983) work, *the Reflective Practitioner*. As an ethicist, she looked "for the moral dimension to any case or situation," and "in my own thinking and in my own practice, I go back and forth between a principle-based approach and a virtue-based, character-based approach . . . I try to talk about the virtues that the ministry needs . . . and the virtues they need to cultivate. But then we also talk about what to do [in certain situations] and why" (Foster et al., 2006, p. 310). All three types of apprenticeship—intellectual, hands-on, and identity formation—are evident in Blodgett's description of her teaching.

Law

In law, Sullivan, Colby, Wegner, Bond, and Shulman (2007) found that legal analysis, practical skill, and professional identity characterized legal education. The researchers found that the signature pedagogy—the case–dialogue method—was so heavily emphasized that other aspects of the students' legal education were neglected. Two examples of "shadow pedagogy" (p. 57) emerged in the study: first, a focus on clients was conspicuously absent and, second, students and some faculty were concerned that the study of ethics within the context of the law lacked "ethical substance" (p. 57).

Researchers recommended a more integrated approach that would tie the purposes of the profession of law with professional identity formation. An increased emphasis in these areas would foster student self-reflection and hopefully help the student become increasingly self-directive as he or she develops a sense of professional ethos (Sullivan et al., 2007).

Engineering

". . . [P]rofessional schools are and should be complex organizations for initiating the next generation of practitioners into the important dimensions of the expertise that defines a given profession" (Sheppard, Macatangay, Colby, & Sullivan, 2009, p. 189). In engineering, study results revealed that although professors were very strong in helping students integrate complex knowledge, more attention was needed to help students integrate their knowledge, skills, and identity as *developing professionals.* Faculty members were charged with changing their paradigmatic view from one of seeing students in seats in classrooms, to seeing young professionals ready to assume their soon-to-be acquired professional roles (Sheppard et al., 2009). The researchers believed that the changes ahead for faculty would be daunting, yet possible. A more comprehensive understanding of integrated learning, along with an intentional focus on professional identity and formation, would bring faculty to a point where they could more ably influence students' entry into the professional world (Sheppard et al., 2009).

Medicine

On November 11, 2009, the Carnegie Foundation for the Advancement of Teaching announced the findings of the last *Preparation for the Professions* study entitled *Educating Physicians: A Call for Reform* (The Carnegie Foundation for the Advancement of Teaching, 2009a). The four key recommendations for improvement in medical education were:

1. More tightly integrate knowledge and experience
2. Create habits of inquiry and improvement
3. Standardize learning outcomes and individualize the learning process
4. Focus on professional identity formation

The results are no surprise given previous study findings in the Carnegie Foundation's *Preparation for the Professions* series. However, in terms of teaching ethics and professionalism, medicine has already been deeply engaged in conversations about professional development because of significant research findings regarding medical professionalism and recent revisions in medical school accreditation criteria that have been in place for nearly a decade.

Papadakis and colleagues (2005) found, in a case-controlled study of state medical boards and medical school graduates, that students who were disciplined for unprofessional behavior in medical school were strongly associated with disciplinary action among practicing physicians by medical boards. The strongest association was with students who were described as "irresponsible or as having diminished ability to improve their behavior" (p. 2673).

Additional disturbing findings indicate the development of professionalism and ethical development may be stifled or even decline throughout the medical education curriculum. Patenaude, Niyonsenga, and Fafard (2003) reported that a leveling or even a decline occurred in moral development during the first three years of medical students' education. The studies by Papadakis et al. (2005) and Paternaude et al. (2003) raise concerns about the need to inculcate professional values during medical school, and the kinds of actions that should be taken when ethical or behavioral issues arise in the academic setting.

Though documents from both the American Medical Association and the American College of Physicians advocate for educating physicians in ethical behavior and professionalism (Doukas, 2003), a significant change occurred in the early 2000's when the Accreditation Council of Graduate Medical Education (ACGME; 2009a, 2009b) instituted competencies specific to professionalism (Doukas, 2003). Because accreditation standards are the means by which residency sites are evaluated, medical schools consider compliance with the ACGME competencies to be crucial. Further, ACGME's outcomes-based assessment approach has increased the available data on medical professionalism and correspondingly added to the current literature. The ACGME competencies appear in Table 6-1.

Nursing

Benner et al. (2010) noted six recommendations for change in how educators think about and design education, based on the work influenced by the Carnegie Foundation

---

Table 6-1   ACGME General Competencies for Professionalism

Residents must demonstrate a commitment to carrying out professional responsibilities and an adherence to ethical principles. Residents are expected to demonstrate:
- compassion, integrity, and respect for others;
- responsiveness to patient needs that supersedes self-interest;
- respect for patient privacy and autonomy;
- accountability to patients, society, and the profession; and
- sensitivity and responsiveness to a diverse patient population, including but not limited to diversity in gender, age, culture, race, religion, disabilities, and sexual orientation.

for the Advancement of Teaching National Study of Nursing Education (p. 390). Five of these recommendations focused on various pedagogical and curricular initiatives, with the sixth recommendation calling for educators to think more transformatively about professional identity formation.

Regarding the recommendation about formation, Benner et al. (2010) asked educators to move away from the notion of *socialization* and *role-taking* and instead focus on *formation*. Such a paradigm shift is both understandable, yet potentially difficult to change. Benner and others have introduced new words to our vocabulary: ethical comportment, formation, apprenticeship—and it is in the hands of nurse educators to understand, define, and operationalize these terms in basic nursing programs. Porter-O'Grady (2009) makes the case that we need to relanguage how we think about the transformation from accepted nursing student to the graduating nurse. We will need to pay close attention to how things are done, what language we use, and the most effective ways to help the discipline grow in order for students to see themselves large enough to make the changes ahead.

UNDERSTANDING STUDENTS IN THE PROFESSIONS: COMMON GROUND

From both a social–cognitive viewpoint and a moral psychology perspective, new research advances offer insights about people within and about to enter professional education. An upturn in interdisciplinary research within the last decade reflects "meta-theoretical perspectives on person-context transaction that unify the work of personality, social and developmental researchers" (Narvaez & Lapsley, 2009, p. 441). Harvard Business School's leadership, ethics, and corporate responsibility initiative (Piper, Gentile, & Parks, 1993) and new developments with the big five personality traits research (McAdams, 2009) form a backdrop in which to better understand the students who are being transformed into professionals.

The Harvard Business School Study— A Constructivist–Developmental Approach

Co-author Sharon Daloz Parks of *Can Ethics Be Taught?* (Piper et al., 1993) wrote, "Empirical evidence demonstrating the importance of moral education in the young adult years has been charted across the last decade and a half . . . and together with insights gained from constructive–developmental learning theory and our own study at the Harvard Business School, strongly suggests that moral development can continue into adulthood, and that particularly dramatic changes can occur in young adulthood in the context of professional school education" (Parks, 1993, p. 13). Parks' extensive prestudy assessment of students entering the Harvard Business School when the ethics, leadership, and corporate responsibility initiative gives insight into students entering professional programs.

These Harvard MBA students—average age, 26—were assessed with two initial assumptions in mind: that all humans seek meaning of the whole, not of the mundane, and that human beings will act in such a way that they can be part of what is perceived to be ultimately true, trustworthy, and dependable (Parks, 1993). Based on her earlier research, Parks expected the students to demonstrate critical, self-aware systemic thought and have a significant measure of inner dependence in the way in which they made meaning of their environments.

As Parks tells the story, a few of her seasoned Harvard Business School faculty colleagues offered an alternate hypothesis—that many of these students might actually be "younger" and "more dependent on authorities and contexts outside the self than one might assume" (p. 23). Parks had identified the two ends of the spectrum in her study as *reflective–personal* and *critical–systemic*. Her colleagues suggested that she would likely find more of the students situated at the *reflective–personal* end of the spectrum. As it turned out, her colleagues were correct.

Overall, Parks found that "without an initiation to critical reflection upon self and upon the systemic complexity and ambiguity these students will be expected to manage, we expect that many of them will continue to subscribe to whatever conventional ethos prevails" (p. 30)—as long as it is successful for them. Specifically, Parks saw that, as a whole, these students were caught up in a flow of success that kept them from experiencing adversity or cognitive dissonance; perceived business as a game, and interpreted morality in entirely interpersonal and private ways (Parks, 1993).

What did this mean for the teachers? Faculty needed to intentionally guide students toward critical–systemic thought, help them recognize and tolerate complexity and ambiguity, and actively engage diverse perspectives (Parks, 1993). The students' heretofore unexamined lives proved to be a disadvantage, leaving them more vulnerable than expected.

In Parks' more recent work (2000), she presents a counterpoint: No matter what the curriculum for ethical reflection will be, it is not compelling in the young adult imagination unless it corresponds with students' perceived requirements of the profession because young adults believe they will be asked to practice it. What then takes place when the student is unfamiliar with the content and purpose of the profession? Further, what occurs when neither the educators nor the institution effectively commensurates the norms of the profession?

The answer seems to rest in the notion of processing, not preaching. According to Parks (2000), every major era or stage in the life span is marked by its own way of making meaning. The sequence is: "(1) becoming critically aware of one's own composing of reality; (2) self-consciously participating in an ongoing dialogue toward truth, (3) cultivating a capacity to respond—to act—in ways that are satisfying and just" (p. 6).

Parks' (2000) social–cognitive model of young adult development captures what she found in her research regarding persons ages 17 to 30. Three domains—*knowing, dependence,* and *community*—that occur in *adolescence/conventional, young adult,* and *tested adult* stages are outlined in Table 6-2. For Parks (2000), it is imperative that those who commit to "recognize and sponsor adult meaning making" (Parks, 2000, p. 69) (i.e., teachers and mentors of young adults) also understand these needs, stages, and meaning. She is particularly attuned to the meaning-making of young adults in academic settings: "Developments in intellectual awareness naturally set in motion a reordering of one's sense of person and space . . . The evolution of meaning occurs in the dance of being affected in one's world coupled with evolving cognitive power" (p. 72).

Parks (2000) described the first of the three periods as *adolescent/conventional* with young persons being authority-bound and moving quickly into unqualified relativism (p. 69), terms understood from the classic works of Piaget, Erikson, and Perry. The *adolescent/conventional* young person is dependent/counterdependent in terms of affective development, vacillating between distancing oneself from authority and actively seeking it. Finally, for the *adolescent/conventional* person, community is identified by "conformity to cultural norms and interests" (Parks, 2000, p. 92), with movement toward a more diffuse understanding of community as unqualified relativism becomes a more prominent consideration in the young person's world.

Perry's (1970) work in intellectual development led Parks (2000) to call the form of knowing in the next period, *young adult*—a period of *probing commitment (ideological),* reflecting the change that occurs when the pros and cons of unbridled relativism finally move the young person to seriously consider some form of commitment. As Parks said, young adults explore many forms of truth during this time, influenced by a growing repertoire of experiences with themselves and their world (Parks, 2000).

Table 6-2   Ways of Knowing, Dependence, and Community for Young Adults

	Adolescent/conventional	Young adult	Tested adult
Knowing	Authority-bound → Unqualified relativism	Probing commitment	Tested commitment
Dependence	Dependent/counterdependent	Fragile inner dependence	Confident inner dependence
Community	Diffuse understanding	Appreciates the mentoring community	Self-selected class/group

Adapted from Parks, S. D. (2000). *Big questions, worthy dreams: Mentoring young adults in their search for meaning, purpose and faith.* San Francisco: Jossey-Bass.

A fragile sense of inner dependence (Parks, 2000) occurs during this period, when the young adult discovers his or her own voice and includes oneself as a part of the domain of authority (Parks, 2000). As Parks (2000) reported, "Here a person begins to listen within, with a new respect and trust for the truth of his or her 'own insides'" (p. 78). In terms of the sense of belonging or community, the young person finds themself seeking and appreciating the mentoring community (Parks, 2000, p. 91). The power of the mentoring relationship is that it helps anchor the young person's vision of the potential self (Parks, 2000). "It is the combination of the emerging developmental stance of the young adult with the challenge and encouragement of the mentor, grounded in the experience of a compatible social group, *that ignites the transforming power of the young adult era* [emphasis added]" (Parks, 2000, p. 93).

The third stage in Parks' model is titled *tested adult*, and includes *tested commitment* in forms of knowing, confident inner dependence, and self-selected class/group as the community. This category constitutes an adult category, as "*adult* connotes one's having achieved the composition of the critically aware self, with its attendant responsibility for the self. The qualifier *young* connotes the ambivalent exploratory, wary, tentative, and dependent quality that is manifest in early adulthood" (p. 70).

Parks (2000) viewed the professions and professional education as necessary contributions to the vitality of our collective common life—a consciousness of the common experience. She asserted that the sense of calling associated with the professions is its greatest strength and the calling of the professions invokes the passion and commitment that otherwise cannot be captured (Parks, 2000). The transformational nature of one's calling to become a nurse, a doctor, or a lawyer elevates the new professional self and profession to the level of the common good. Professional education helps with "meaning-making" (p. 175) and becomes the basis for making critical choices (Parks, 2000).

Building on the Big Five: An Integrative Model of Personality

Though the following example is largely a psychological and personality-based perspective, it is the developmental scholars (Erikson, Kohlberg, and others) who have confirmed that *moral identity* and *agency* continue to develop post-school age (Lapsley, 1996). These findings are helpful to those who mentor persons in their meaning-making as they learn their chosen profession.

Over the last 10 years it has become clear that personality traits, often referred to as dispositions, are now thought to be exceedingly stable over time. These become the bottom row of building blocks on which personalities operate (see Table 6-3). The most well-known understanding of these dispositions is referred to as the "Big Five" (Fig. 6-1), which divide traits into the categories of "extraversion (vs introversion), neuroticism (vs emotional stability), conscientiousness, agreeableness, and openness to experience" (McAdams, 2009, p. 13). Although dispositional traits do not tell the entire story, they do represent an important starting point in

Table 6-3   Fundamental Principles for an Integrative Science of Personality

An individual's unique variation on the general evolutionary design for human nature is expressed as a developing pattern of:
- Dispositional traits (also known as the "Big Five" model of personality)
- Characteristic adaptations
- Self-defining life narratives
- Situations within the cultural and social context

Source: Adapted from McAdams & Pals, 2006.

understanding human behavior. Dispositional traits form the basis for a number of preemployment instruments designed to achieve the best fit between potential employee and employer. The Healthcare Selection Inventory (HSI), one such pre-employment screening tool, can account for approximately 10% of the variance in hiring success This instrument is endorsed by the American Hospital Association and used in more than 500 hundred hospitals nationwide (M. Wiersma, personal communication, November 14, 2009).

Figure 6-1   The "Big Five" dispositions (McAdams, 2009).

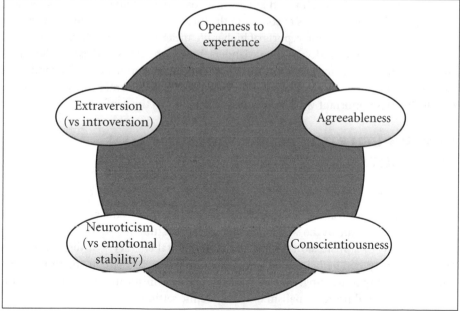

McAdams and Pals (2006), leading researchers in the area of the "Big Five," have used what is known about these stable dispositional traits to further develop an integrative model of personality. The integrative model is composed of: "(1) an individual's unique variation on general evolutionary design for human nature, which is (2) experienced as a pattern of dispositional traits, (3) characteristic adaptations, and (4) self-defining life narratives, which are (5) situated complexly in social contexts and culture" (McAdams, 2009, p. 12). A schematic of this model appears in Table 6-3.

Such an integrative model of personality can be helpful in understanding and mentoring young adults as they progress in their professional education because findings about stable human dispositions have implications for prosocial behavior and behavioral understanding. For instance, "high scores on the dispositional traits of conscientiousness and agreeableness have been linked to pro-social behavior, commitment to societal institutions, honesty, integrity and fewer instances of violating moral norms" (McAdams, 2009, p. 24). At least moderately high levels of openness to experience appear to be a prerequisite for valuing tolerance and diversity in society. "Of course, high scores on these traits do not guarantee these behavioral correlates for every case; empirical findings in psychology are almost always probabilistic. But all other things being equal, high levels of conscientiousness, agreeableness and openness to experience lay the foundation for a moral personality" (McAdams, 2009, p. 24).

It is the developmental aspect of the integrative model of personality that holds the most promise for influencing young professionals. McAdams (2009) finds that *characteristic adaptations* that are most instrumental in shaping morality are personal goals and projects. Research has shown that personal goals focused on caring for others and making positive contributions to society in the future are often associated with greater psychological well-being and reports of higher life meaning (Bauer & McAdams, 2004; Emmons, 2009; Kasser & Ryan, 1996). Understanding the traits and exactly how they are stable and working in mentoring environments to communicate understanding as well as opportunities for change based on contextual and cultural influences (Lapsley & Hill, 2009) is important work in mentoring students in the professions.

HOW SHOULD ETHICS AND PROFESSIONALISM BE TAUGHT?

Five Themes

Work within other professions can effectively inform nursing education and practice. Nursing is not unique in the way in which it prepares students for the profession. An understanding of a professional *ethos*, the fundamental character or disposition of a group or society, can be helpful in more intentionally crafting the formation of professional identity in nursing. Five general themes communicate useful direction for teaching ethics and professionalism in the academic setting.

Explicitly

Aspects of curricula that focus on professionalism and ethics must be explicit and intentional (Patenaude et al., 2003) because behavior in a professional program is strongly associated with the presence or absence of professional behaviors in subsequent practice (Papadakis et al., 2005). Students generally respond well to ethics education, particularly when it is situated in clinical and small group contexts (Goldie, Dowie, Cotton, & Morrison, 2007; Roberts, Hammond, Geppert, & Warner, 2004; Shrank, Reed, & Jernstedt, 2004). Self-reflection is extremely critical and should be incorporated in pedagogically grounded ways (Haidet, 2008). Finally, the institution is the instrument for communicating ethics and professionalism, perhaps even more than the professor or the students (Haidet, 2008; Holtman, 2008). An educational ethos that embraces rigorous analysis and informed imagination regarding ethics and professionalism will explicitly communicate these values to the entire learning community.

Knowledgeably

It has been said that the biggest change in higher education within the last 10 years *is the students themselves.* As Parks (2000) commented, without student ownership of the requirements of the profession—as the profession sees them, not as the student imagines them to be—no amount of ethical reflection will be effective. Faculty will be more effective if they use what is known about students to help them develop their own *personal professional ideal* and their *social ideal* or expected behaviors by the profession. Educators can craft curricula not only about bringing students forward and inculcating a balance between the role as the student and the role as the individual moral agent, but also about the discipline. Nurse professionals are mindful of not only the influence of peers and peer values, and of the human tendency to stay with a conventional ethos if it continues to work (Parks, 1993), but also the restriction that conventional ethos places on one when one is morally compelled to resist it. Meaning-making is an interactive process and thus is dependent on and stimulated by the conditions of the environment. It is also a process of seeking order, pattern, and significance (Parks, 2000). A more knowledge-driven and intentional educational approach is needed in order to be *compelling enough* for students to own their professional ideals and to respect and work within a professional ethos.

Dialogically

One of the pervasive problems of professional education discovered in the Carnegie study, *Preparations for the Professions* (The Carnegie Foundation for the Advancement of Teaching, 2009b) is the narrowing of rational discourse to simple rational calculations, formal criteria reasoning, "rule in/rule out," and cost–benefit analyses (Benner, Tanner, & Chesla, 2009, p. 392). These researchers advocate a more dialogical approach to integrating theory and practice, in part because nursing is a socially embedded practice (Benner, et al., 2009). Dialogical discourse is the "systematic study of dialogues in which two parties exchange arguments over a central claim" (Keiff, 2009). Benner, Tanner, and Chesla (2009) argue that the rich, relational nature of nursing practice cannot be falsely reduced to mere calculations. To learn nursing, it must be a relational, dialogical process that embeds the nuances of a very complex practice. Creating learning environments that use dialogical pedagogy as a central theme is essential for nursing education. Yet, given the nature of the profession and the speed at which these students are educated, such an approach is difficult to fully convey the discipline to those entering the field.

Contextually as Legitimate Peripheral Participation

It is not unusual for nurses with rich practice experiences who consistently put patients' needs first to come to the educational setting and try to transfer this same approach to teaching students who seek to provide the best education (read: patient care) possible. Because most learning environments in undergraduate nursing programs include multiple students, the premise of providing the "best possible care" (or, in this case the best possible individualized education) is not possible. Using the same patient care paradigm is not a practical one; there is no way that nursing education can totally be a one-to-one endeavor. Yet educators, with no viable alternative model—new and seasoned alike—may gravitate toward the individualized model for students. Lave and Wenger (1991) suggest a different model: one where legitimate peripheral participation is understood as a viewpoint on learning. This idea situates *learning as an integral and inseparable aspect of social practice*, and looks at *practice, person*, and *social world* as concepts of interest in this particular analysis of learning. Thus, the student becomes a learner through practice in both the personal and social elements.

However, legitimate peripheral participation is not always an easy transition within a professional program. Ginsburg, Kachan, and Lingard (2005) found that preclerkship (pre-clinical) medical students involved in professional lapses used both dissociation and engagement in making meaning of their experiences. Ginsburg and her colleagues posited that students' past experiences being center stage in the academic classroom prior to professional education did not serve them well in adapting to the professional school environment. "Students' awkward transference of an egocentric classroom attitude which expects that all events will be tailored to their learning, makes them uneasy with their role in a complex, situated learning setting in which their interests are in competition with a myriad of others" (Ginsburg et al., 2005, p. 18). Actively changing the paradigm for faculty and students within professional educational settings from one where the student is in the center of the circle, to one where the discipline becomes the central focus of the educational process may substantially help students' transition into a new, critical–systemic perspective that more readily accepts a professional ethos.

Transformationally

Finally, the sights of those who plan and deliver professional education, should be focused on helping transform the student from a naïve consumer to a learned professional. *Telos*—the purpose that nurse professionals move toward and the ideal to achieve—is important at every step in the process. If the students are told that the goal is for them to pass the pharmacology test, then they adopt that as the goal. However, if the larger goal of all involved is to help the student transform into a professional who has good character, who is knowledgeable, and who does good work in practice, then that too can be conveyed from the very beginning of the educational process.

As McAdams (2009) noted, personal goals and aspirations are the most powerful characteristic adaptations that occur in the integrated model of personality. Those involved in "recognizing and sponsoring meaning-making" (Parks, 2000) for professional students must set the course, precisely and clearly, for students to transform into the professionals demanded by best practices in the profession. A transformational mindset is central for students, faculty, and administration because all participate in the social practice of the professions.

After all, effective educators engage in their discipline because they have found some degree of transcendent meaning in the work that they do (Palmer, 1998). Moving students to apply critical–systemic thought, enabling them to tolerate complexity and ambiguity in the service of composing new frames for good nursing and good practice, encouraging active and productive student leadership, and cultivating a new imagination in the context of diverse perspectives are noble goals for those who help in the meaning-making process for those who seek professional membership.

REFERENCES

Accreditation Council of Graduate Medical Education. (2009a). *Common program requirements.* Available online at: http://www.acgme.org/Outcome. Accessed November 15, 2009.

Accreditation Council of Graduate Medical Education. (2009b). *General competencies.* Available online at: http://www.acgme.org/outcome/comp/GeneralCompetenciesStandards21307.pdf. Accessed November 15, 2009.

Bauer, J. J., & McAdams, D. P. (2004). Growth goals, maturity, and well being. *Developmental Psychology, 40*, 114–127.

Benner, P., Sutphen, M., Leonard-Kahn, V., & Day, L. (2008). Formation and everyday ethical comportment. *American Journal of Critical Care, 17*(5), 473–476.

Benner, P., Sutphen, M., Leonard-Kahn, V., & Day, L. (2010). *Educating nurses: A call for radical transformation*. San Francisco: Jossey-Bass and Stanford, CA: Carnegie Foundation for the Advancement of Teaching.

Benner, P., Tanner, C., & Chesla, C. (2009). *Expertise in nursing practice: Caring, clinical judgment, and ethics* (2nd ed.). New York: Springer.

Billings, D. M., & Halstead, J. A. (2009). *Teaching in nursing: A guide for faculty* (3rd ed.). Philadelphia: Saunders Co.

The Carnegie Foundation for the Advancement of Teaching. (2009a). *Educating physicians: A call for reform*. Available online at: http://www.carnegiefoundation.org/carnegie-connections /whats-happening/standing-room-only. Accessed November 15, 2009.

The Carnegie Foundation for the Advancement of Teaching. (2009b). *Preparing the professions*. Available online at: http://www.carnegiefoundation.org/previous-work/professional-graduate-education. Accessed December 12, 2009.

The Carnegie Foundation for the Advancement of Teaching. (2009c). *Study of nursing education*. Available online at: http://www.carnegiefoundation.org/nursing-education. Accessed November 15, 2009.

Doukas, D. J. (2003). Where is the virtue in professionalism? *Cambridge Quarterly of Healthcare Ethics, 12*, 147–154.

Emmons, R. A. (2009). Greatest of the virtues? Gratitude and the grateful personality. In D. Narvaez & D. K. Lapsley (Eds.), *Personality, identity and character: Explorations in moral psychology* (pp. 256–270). New York: Cambridge University Press.

Foster, C. R., Dahill, L. E., Golemon, L. A., & Tolentino, B. W. (2006). *Educating clergy: Teaching practices and pastoral imagination*. San Francisco:Jossey-Bass and Stanford, CA: Carnegie Foundation for the Advancement of Teaching.

Ginsburg, S., Kachan, N., & Lingard, L. (2005). Before the white coat: Perceptions of professional lapses in the pre-clerkship. *Medical Education, 39*, 12–19.

Goldie, J., Dowie, A., Cotton, P., & Morrison, J. (2007). Teaching professionalism in the early years of a medical curriculum: A qualitative study. *Medical Education, 41*, 610–616.

Haidet, P. (2008). Where we're headed: A new wave of scholarship on educating medical professionalism. *Journal of General Internal Medicine, 23*(7), 1118–1119.

Holtman, M. C. (2008). A theoretical sketch of medical professionalism as a normative complex. *Advances in Health Science Education, 13*, 233–245.

Kasser, T., & Ryan, R. M. (1996). Further examining the American dream: Well-being correlates of intrinsic and extrinsic goals. *Personality and Social Psychology Bulletin, 22*, 281–288.

Keiff, L. (2009). Dialogical logic. In E. N. Zalta (Ed.), *The Stanford encyclopedia of philosophy* Available online at: http://plato.stanford.edu/archives/sum2009/entries/logic-dialogical. Accessed November 20, 2009.

Lapsley, D. K. (1996). *Moral psychology*. Boulder, CO: Westview Press.

Lapsley, D. K., & Hill, P. K. (2009). The development of moral personality. In D. Narvaez & D. K. Lapsley (Eds.), *Personality, identity and character: Explorations in moral psychology* (pp. 185–213). New York: Cambridge University Press.

Lave, J., & Wenger, E. (1991). *Situated learning: Legitimate peripheral participation*. New York: Cambridge University Press.

McAdams, D. P. (2009). The moral personality. In D. Narvaez & D. K. Lapsley (Eds.), *Personality, identity and character: Explorations in moral psychology* (pp. 11–29). New York: Cambridge University Press.

McAdams, D. P., & Pals, J. L. (2006). A new Big Five: Fundamental principles for an integrative science of personality. *American Psychologist, 61,* 204–217.

Narvaez, D., & Lapsley, D. (2009). *Personality, identity and character: Explorations in moral psychology.* New York: Cambridge University Press.

O'Connor, S. J. (2007). Developing professional habitus: A Bernsteinian analysis of the modern nurse apprenticeship. *Nurse Education Today, 27,* 748–754.

Palmer, P. (1998). *The courage to teach: Exploring the inner landscape of a teacher's life.* San Francisco: Jossey-Bass.

Papadakis, M. A., Teherani, A., Banach, M. A., Knettler, T. R., Rattner, S. L., Stern, D. T., et al. (2005). Disciplinary action by medical boards and prior behavior in medical school. *New England Journal of Medicine, 353*(25), 2673–2682.

Parks, S. D. (1993). Is it too late? Young adults and the formation of professional ethics. In T. R. Piper, M. C. Gentile, & S. D. Parks (Eds.), *Can ethics be taught? Perspectives, challenges, and approaches at Harvard Business School* (pp. 13–72). Boston: Harvard Business School.

Parks, S. D. (2000). *Big questions, worthy dreams: Mentoring young adults in their search for meaning, purpose and faith.* San Francisco: Jossey-Bass.

Patenaude, J., Niyonsenga, T., & Fafard, D. (2003). Changes in students' moral development during medical school: A cohort study. *Canadian Medical Association Journal, 168*(7), 840–844.

Perry, W. G. (1970). *Forms of intellectual and ethical development in the college years: A scheme.* New York: Holt, Rinehart and Winston.

Piper, T. R., Gentile, M. C., & Parks, S. D. (1993). *Can ethics be taught? Perspectives, challenges, and approaches at Harvard Business School.* Boston: Harvard Business School.

Porter-O'Grady, T. (2009). *Healthcare 2010 and Beyond.* Lessons from Legends Series, University of Kansas School of Nursing, November 6, 2009.

Roberts, L. W., Hammond, K. A., Geppert, C. M., & Warner, T. D. (2004). The positive role model of professionalism and ethics training in medical education: A comparison of medical student and resident perspectives. *Academic Psychiatry, 28*(3), 170–182.

Schon, D. (1983). *The reflective practitioner: How professionals think in action.* New York: Basic Books.

Sheppard, S. D., Macatangay, K., Colby, A., & Sullivan, W. M. (2009). *Educating engineers: Designing the future of the field.* San Francisco: Jossey-Bass and Stanford, CA: The Carnegie Foundation for the Advancement of Teaching.

Shrank, W. H., Reed, V. A., & Jernstedt, G. C. (2004). Fostering professionalism in medical education. *Journal of General Internal Medicine, 19,* 887–892.

Smith, K. V., & Godfrey, N. S. (2002). Being a good nurse and doing the right thing: A qualitative study. *Nursing Ethics, 9*(3), 301–312.

Sullivan, W. M., Colby, A., Wegner, J. W., Bond, L., & Shulman, L. S. (2007). *Educating lawyers: Preparation for the profession of law.* San Francisco: John Wiley & Sons.

CHAPTER 7

Measuring Professionalism

Professional practice is predominantly
a moral enterprise.

—M. J. Bebeau, 2002

Well planned and implemented curricula are necessary but not sufficient for quality professional education. Evaluation is essential for determining if curricula are effective in facilitating students' professional development. Measuring professional growth as students progress through the program and professional life after graduation are not easy tasks for any discipline, and nursing is no exception (Lynch, Surdyk, & Eiser, 2004).

The first section of this chapter presents the results of a review of the extensive work that has been done toward developing methods for evaluating professionalism. The following sections explore evaluative methods that are conceptually consistent with the proposed Framework for Nurse Professionals (FrNPs) and Stairstep Model of Professional Transformation, and suggest further direction for professional evaluation.

STRUCTURING PROFESSIONALISM

Professionalism is a construct that can be measured either *directly* as a global term, or *indirectly* as traits that are identified as part of professionalism. For example, honesty, compassion, open-mindedness, integrity, and punctuality are clearly related to professionalism and can be measured. Veloski, Fields, Boex, and Blank (2005) in their literature review of instruments that measure professionalism during 1982 to 2002, reported that over 114 different concepts had been used as indirect indicators of professionalism.

Instruments may measure either *psychological* variables and individual's perceptions of traits, virtues, and attitudes, or *sociological* variables of how one is perceived by others. Although qualitative evaluation more closely aligns with the psychological paradigm and quantitative inquiry with the sociological paradigm, instrumentation for either may be purely qualitative or quantitative or a combination of the two.

Clinical performance has always been highly valued in the assessment of professional development in any applied discipline but is notoriously difficult to evaluate. Faculty express concern over too few parameters to assess, too many students in the clinical setting to properly evaluate, and a belief that testing knowledge is the primary method of assessing student performance in the nursing program. Despite these challenges, clinical remains the ultimate means to evaluate student capacities to do the work of nursing because it is where professionalism is put into practice. Laboratory scenarios, classroom tests, and simulations are helpful tools but do not take the place of actual clinical experience and evaluation.

A good deal of evaluation of curricula and student progress occurs in most nursing programs. Faculty evaluate through *standardized* and *specific* methods. Often, faculty develop evaluation tools that assess student skills, knowledge, and professional behaviors that are designed for evaluating success in meeting program specific unit, course, or curricular objectives and outcomes. Standardized assessment instruments like student satisfaction and knowledge development over the curricula, are also widely used. Together the standardized and specific instruments measure an array of perceptions, qualities, behaviors, and observations made by the various people who interact and observe students.

Traditional evaluation of student professionalism, skills, and knowledge has been performed using the *perceptions* of educators. However, there is a growing body of knowledge that multiple sources of information improve evaluation and may also improve student professional development. A number of different observers in addition to traditional faculty and self-evaluation can be used (Table 7-1). Peer review is less frequently used but can be a valuable method of evaluation. Medicine and other disciplines have moved in the direction of using more clinical evaluation by peers (Kovach, Resch, & Verhuist, 2009; Quiantance, Arnold, & Thompson, 2008). Work with peer evaluations has also raised educator awareness of the challenges to reliability and objectivity that nontraditional evaluator-observers and particularly peer evaluation bring (Arnold, 2002; Kovach et al., 2009). Use of evaluators from a variety of sources has the potential for great benefit but, if not done with care, could potentially have negative effects. The use of multiple sources for student evaluation should be prefaced with a caveat that methods be carefully developed and considered in light of limitations.

Table 7-1 Types of Measurement of Professionalism

Qualitative	Quantitative
Reflection	Surveys/questionnaires
Portfolios	Behavioral/field observations
Journaling	Postgraduation follow-up
Evaluation: clinical, lab, and classroom	Evaluation: clinical, lab, and classroom

PROFESSIONALISM AND ETHICS

Ethics

No matter what direction the conceptualization of professionalism takes, whether it be by psychological or sociological, all conceptualizations are based on an ethical foundation (McAdams, 2009; Rogers, Mentkowski, Hart, & Minik, 2001). There is also a greater synthesis of ethics with other disciplines' scopes of interest. Recent work in psychology confirms that moral developmental theory, cognitive psychology, and developmental psychology are closely related and are in need of contextualization within the human personality (Narvaez & Lapsley, 2009).

The recognition that a strong relationship exists among professionalism, human sciences, and ethics and that there is a need for a more integrated and contextualized understanding of professionalism appears to be a watershed phenomenon that has emerged across all disciplines (Fleischmann, 2004; Lemonidou, Papathanassoglou, Giannakopoulou, Patiraki, & Papadatou, 2004; Pellegrino, 2006). Evaluation of professionalism is an evaluation of ethical development. Scholarly work in ethics has been directed at moral development in general and not specifically to professional development. The most researched area of ethics by far has been moral reasoning or decision making (Bebeau, 2002; Rogers et al., 2001). Work in moral development by Kohlberg, Lovinger, Gilligan, and Rest, among others, have helped to broaden and structure ethical responsiveness to more than just reasoning.

Moral Theorists

Professionalism is often evaluated through instruments that measure moral development. Before discussing specific instruments, three theorists who have influenced professionalism through the moral development theory deserve brief mention.

Kohlberg

Kohlberg's theory of moral development is widely known and forms the conceptual basis for a number ethical measurement instruments used in professional and ethical education evaluation. Kohlberg claimed that ethical development occurs at three stages: preconventional, conventional, and, the most advanced form of ethical thinking, the postconventional stage. People who function at the preconventional level make decisions from fear or potential punishment. The conventional level that corresponds to the sociological paradigm is evidenced when an individual bases decisions on rules, norms, and expectations. The individual who makes decisions at the postconventional stage is able to individualize and contextualize decision making and base decisions on fairness to others rather than from fear of punishment or by following rules (Kohlberg, 1981; Rogers et al., 2001). Kohlberg was a student of R. M. Hare and the postconventional stage appears to approach what Hare called "critical level" of moral reasoning in which universalizability is used to determine best decisions (Hare, 1989). Universalizability is a logical way of thinking about others and is close conceptually to other ways that justice is operationalized. Justice is also the evident moral concept in what many call golden rule thinking—the consequential tradition of everyone counts for one—and Kant's categorical imperative. Individuals who use these logical thought processes have the ability to step outside themselves and to make choices and act based on fairness through granting equal moral agency to others. They are able to treat others with the same ethical sensitivity and respect that they would treat themselves if they were to exchange places (Crigger, 1994; Hare, 1989).

Not all people, according to Kohlberg, will develop their postconventional abilities. Cultural norms or societies in which the individual moral agent is embedded may overrule the ability to see each person's perspective as equal. For example, in war the soldier must adhere to the convention and commitment to that of a soldier and view others as enemies. Even today, sects of some world religions believe and act on doctrines that view people outside their religion as undeserving of the same moral respect as they themselves are due because they do not embrace the religious devotees' faith. Then, the cultural norms such as not to lie or kill apply only to those within the faith, and those outside the faith are not granted equal moral agency and therefore lying to a nonbeliever or killing a nonbeliever is not morally wrong.

Previous research to determine the ethical development level of nurses based on the Kohlbergian theory has been disheartening. A meta-analysis of nine studies conducted in four different developed nations by Dierckx de Casterle, Izumi, Godfrey, and Denhaerynck (2008) indicated that nurses generally were conformist and functioned at the conventional level of moral development. The researchers concluded that development at postconventional was present in only a few expert nurses that were assessed. Although meeting the professional social expectations—following rules and meeting expectations are good, there are certain times and situations when nurses should function beyond the conventional and make decisions through universalizing. The researchers encouraged nurse educators, leaders, and researchers to advance ethical development in nurses and the profession and find ways to promote growth toward educating nurses to think beyond conventional levels.

Gilligan

Gilligan's work from the scientific discipline sparked what one author calls "the Kohlberg-Gilligan debate" (Gastmans, 2006). Gilligan's theory of moral development (1982) was developed through qualitative research on women who had undergone abortions. Based on her work, Gilligan believed that development of men and women differed and that women used a relational ethic of caring rather than one of justice as suggested by Kohlberg. This relational ethic has a more significant role to play in the motivation and justification of ethical decisions and actions.

Rest

Rest (1986), a highly influential theorist, advanced a model of moral development that has been widely used in ethics education and professional ethics in many disciplines. The model is called a framework of *moral responsiveness* and is partitioned into four elements: moral judgment, moral sensitivity, moral motivation (values and priority), and moral character (ability of decision-maker to follow through with action). Rest believed that, although each of the four elements was closely related to the others, they were different enough to be measured separately. Rest's framework promoted development of instruments that specifically measure each of the four concepts.

Ethical Measures Using Rest's Framework of Moral Responsiveness

This section is not designed to give specific instrument qualities, like reliability scores or development, or to provide a comprehensive review of all instruments available, but rather to provide the reader with general information about a few of the well-established instruments available for measuring each of the four elements.

Moral Reasoning

Moral reasoning is the ability to justify moral decisions through logic and reason. Although moral reasoning and decision making are often presented as distinct from professionalism, there appears to be a significant relationship between moral reasoning and moral performance in clinical settings (Baldwin & Self, 2006). Previous research also suggests that levels of moral development relate to clinical performance in students. Studies that assess the progression of moral development have been most extensive with medical students and have yielded conflicting results. Medical education, and particularly when students are in clinical practice settings, suggests that student moral development plateaus or even regresses along the Kohlbergian stages. This "ethical erosion" suggests that professional education may even have a negative impact on moral development (Patenaude, Niyonsenga, & Fafard, 2003) and also implicates forms of hidden curricula, like attitudes of mentors and peers, as the source of moral regression (Baldwin & Self, 2006). Both the *moral judgment interview* (MJI) and the *defining issues test* (DIT) measure moral judgment.

Moral Judgment Interview (MJI)

The MJI, developed by Kohlberg (Colby & Kohlberg, 1987), measures levels of moral decision making and has been extensively developed and assessed with multiple populations. The MJI is used to obtain responses through an interview format that asks subjects to respond to three hypothetical cases and takes around 45 minutes to administer. The MJI requires special training for the test administrator and the cost for administration is considerable. A self-administered questionnaire of the MJI, the sociomoral reasoning measure (SRM) was later developed (Baldwin & Self, 2006) and makes the instrument less costly and more accessible.

Another useful test for moral reasoning measurement is the Defining Issues Test (DIT; Association of American Colleges and Universities [AACU], 2010). Although the DIT is primarily a test of moral reasoning (Lynch et al., 2004) some sources of information reviewed report that this instrument measures both judgment and moral sensitivity. Because the DIT measures two different concepts, further discussion of the instrument is continued in the moral sensitivity section.

Moral Sensitivity

Moral sensitivity is one's ability to interpret situations that are morally relevant and also to be sensitive to reactions and feeling of others (Bebeau, 2002; Rest, 1986). Moral sensitivity, like moral reasoning, has stimulated instrument development (Lynch et al., 2004; Myyry & Helkama, 2002). Instruments that measure moral sensitivity are much less common than instruments that measure moral reasoning and judgment. Most studies that were developed to measure sensitivity were initially conducted on professionals rather than students (Bebeau, 2002) but, more recently, have been used in educational settings. Two instruments, the DIT and the dental ethical sensitivity test are the most developed of the instruments to measure moral awareness and sensitivity.

The Defining Issues Test (DIT)

The DIT is reported to be an instrument that measures moral reasoning and judgment as well as sensitivity to moral situations. This conceptual blending appears to occur in many other instruments that report moral sensitivity and reasoning together.

A review of research studies indicates that the DIT has been used in over 500 different studies (AACU, 2010). The DIT is based on Kohlberg's theory of moral development as the standard of moral progress, and measures sensitivity and reasoning. The DIT is a self-administered quantitative questionnaire that uses six moral dilemmas with responses as ordinal level measurement.

Bebeau (2002) has conducted the most extensive work on the efficacy of the DIT to evaluate ethical development. Bebeau (2002) reviewed 33 studies from five professions to determine the effect that education has on moral reasoning and sensitivity as measured by the DIT. One of the five professions reviewed was nursing and there were conflicting results. Bebeau (2002) reported that nursing had a significant amount of research published on sensitivity and moral reasoning and that the studies overall failed to demonstrate an improvement in moral sensitivity and judgment as students progressed in their educational programs. The more recent nursing studies, Bebeau concluded, were poorly designed and led one to question the validity and reliability of these findings. Of the studies reviewed, two longitudinal studies conducted in the 1990s (Duckett et al., 1992; Duckett et al., 1997) were reported to be well conceptualized and conducted. These larger, earlier longitudinal studies found a significant increase in DIT scores over time in the student nurses studied, suggesting that professional education improved student's moral sensitivity and reasoning.

Overall, Bebeau (2002) concluded that the results of the review of studies in all five disciplines studied as a whole did not demonstrate a significant change in moral judgment in students over time but found that students gained a greater sensitivity to moral issues as they progressed through the educational program. Further, an understanding of moral judgment is important in professional education, but Bebeau claimed that the other components of Rest's four component model were essential to evaluate in professional education so that educators could obtain a more complete picture of professional education and practice.

The Dental Ethical Sensitivity Test

A second instrument, the dental ethical sensitivity test (DEST form A and B), purports to measure sensitivity in dental education students and has been evaluated with extensively developed construct validity (Bebeau, 2002; Bebeau, Rest, & Yamoor, 1985). Other professions have used varied methods to evaluate sensitivity that include role play, video/DVD or audiotape recordings, as well as the more established vignettes with short answers (Lynch et al., 2004).

Sensitivity Measures in Nursing

Bebeau's (2002) evaluation of measures of sensitivity in nursing was correct. A large part of the discipline's effort to develop instrumentation to measure moral development and professionalism has been directed at measuring sensitivity to morally significant situations and the response of others.

One study of nursing students in Finland (Myyry & Helkama, 2002) investigated sensitivity to moral issues and value priorities, thus comparing two of the four concepts of moral responsiveness. The researchers used an established instrument, the Schwartz Value Survey (SVS), but, in addition, developed and used their own instrumentation to measure sensitivity that consisted of presenting a case and using a scoring system that was similar to one developed by Bebeau. No psychometric evaluations are reported by the authors and no specific name is given to the instrument (Schwartz, 1992).

Sensitivity approximates the concept of caring, and caring has been identified by some authors as essential to professionalism and practice in nursing. Swanson (1999), in a comprehensive literature review, reported on seven different instruments used in nursing to measure caring and concluded that most of the instruments were not psychometrically sound. The Coates Caring Efficacy Scale (CES), developed by nurses to measure caring capacity (Coates, 1997; Sadler, 2003), appears to be further from the original intent of sensitivity to ethical situations and is a general measure of caring ability, although it does clearly relate to moral sensitivity.

Moral Motivation

Moral motivation, the third element described in Rest's model, refers to how one prioritizes competing loyalties and desires. Moral values have been of interest to educators for some time because in common sense psychology a moral agent is believed to be motivated by and acts according to the values that he or she holds. In today's pluralistic society, nursing students come into programs with varied values. There are varieties of age, a more equal male to female ratio, more minority students, and an increasing number of students from a variety of religious and cultural backgrounds.

Although some accommodation can be made for students who hold differing values, there are still core values and behaviors that are expected from nurse professionals, like honesty, integrity, loyalty, and cultural sensitivity. The values of a nurse come initially from the sociological paradigm and from common knowledge of nursing—through teachers, other nurses, work settings, and, most importantly, through the expectations of the profession. Essential values are cultivated into a student nurse's professional and personal ideal portraits as they progress through the educational process. These professional values are adopted and become the touchstones for the professional's prioritizing of goals and motivations (Rest, 1986).

Bebeau (2002) links values and motivations closely to identity formation, stating that people hold varying values that may "penetrate" their self understanding to differing degrees. Professional values may differ in cultures quite significantly and even in students from differing disciplines (Thorpe & Loo, 2003; Yeun, Kwon, & Ahn, 2005). For example, a nurse professional may have value conflicts while providing care for a patient who has an elective abortion; the nurse's personal values of faith may be in direct conflict with that patient. Nurse professionals may be strongly compelled to follow his or her commitment to faith rather than uphold a commitment to patient care or vice versa.

Professional and personal values can be both social and personal constructs as evidenced through the two paradigms of professionalism. Therefore, a clear understanding of what constitutes valued ideals, goals, and characteristics for any profession as well as for each individual is needed before value priorities can be understood. Although a number of measures have been developed through other disciplines, the discussion is limited to the literature review findings on nursing. For further information on values instrumentation the reader is referred to Lynch et al. (2004).

Nursing and Research on Values

Rassin Values Scale

Values research in nursing has changed the disciplines' understanding of values. Rassin (2008) studied a group of nurses who had immigrated to Israel from various global locations. Two instruments were used: the Rokeach values survey (RVS)

(Braithwaite & Law, 1985; Rokeach, 1973) and an instrument that measured professional values as developed by the researchers. The researchers reported that professional values varied significantly among the nurses and reasoned that the differences were because of the cultural backgrounds.

The RVS has well-established psychometric properties and is self-administered. Test takers rank the various values in two different areas: instrumentalism and terminal values. Instrumentalism corresponds to personal characteristics like politeness, honesty, or ambition, and terminal values included goal orientation, like family security, social recognition, and happiness.

Schwartz Value Test

Another test that measure values is the Schwartz value test (SVT; 1992). The SVT is conceptually a well developed instrument that measures value priorities based on Schwartz's 11 value types: power, achievement, self-direction, universalism, hedonism, benevolence, tradition, conformity, security, caring, and spirituality. These values can be further divided into whether the respondent has an individualistic or a community interest orientation.

Nurses Professional Values Scale

The nurse professional values scale (NPVS) was reported to be developed from the American Nurses Association code of ethics (1998) and literature pertaining to it by Weis and Schank (2000). The instrument is an ordinal level measurement of eight factors (identified with factor analysis), of which care giving was the highest of the eight value factors. A revised version of the instrument (NPUS-R) was recently introduced (Weis & Schank, 2009).

Moral Character

Moral character, as identified by Rest (1986), is the ability to follow through on a moral plan of action. Moral character, as defined by Rest, comes close to phronesis or practical wisdom and the proper use of virtues, and is the ability of one to conform one's impulses, desires, and actions to promote choices that lead to excellence in practice and build good character. Moral character is the most difficult of the four moral elements to measure because it relies on the actions or outcomes of moral thinking. As with Rest's definition—unlike reasoning and judgment, moral sensitivity, and moral motivation that can be measured through hypothetical case studies, rankings, and attitudes—moral character suggests that one's actions need to be assessed over time.

Is character generally thought of as a behavior or is Rest's interpretation of character different? The word character has a number of different uses that speak to both the *pattern of one's behavior* as Rest and phronesis suggest, but also to the *quality, traits*, and *virtues* of an individual. Research has been conducted and instruments have been developed that define character as traits or virtues but also as a pattern of behavior, each of which is discussed.

Character as Traits or Virtue

There are only a few instruments that measure character and the associated professional virtues or traits. Some traits or virtues that have been measured in current instruments include, for example, attitudes toward trust, deception, caring, emotional intelligence, cynicism, attitudes toward cheating, and social responsibility (Lynch et al., 2004). McAdams (2009) identifies moral personality as the "broad aspect of the human being that is the organization within an individual of his or her unique adjustment to life situations" (p. 12) that is made up of the dispositional traits, character adaptations, and life narratives.

The core or fundamental desired character virtues or traits, when compared by the authors, are similar in nursing, medicine, pharmacy, and dental professionals (Davis, 2002; Elman, Illfelder-Kaye, & Robiner, 2005). When and how are student's traits and virtues contributing to professional development? Do they remain fundamentally stable during the educational process or are they modified by education? Traits are certainly more stable—as is the trait form of virtue—but, through the perspective of virtue ethics, character development traits and virtue traits are modified through experience and education.

Sentence Completion Test

Only one instrument that measures what might be character traits or virtues was identified. The Sentence Completion Test (SCT), used to measure ego development and personality, is a qualitative instrument of 36 sentence stems that are completed by the test taker (Lynch et al., 2004).

Preprofessional Character

Although little research has been reported on the relationship of preprofessional character and successful adaptation to a profession later, two published articles from two nonnursing disciplines suggest that preprofessional personality and character may play an important role in successful professional development.

Coulehan and Williams (2003), recognizing that the medical education system teaches professionalism through both tacit and hidden curriculum and explicit education, advanced an interesting theory of medical students' professional growth. Through observations made over their years in medical education, the physician educators concluded that medical students, when faced with the conflict of tacit and explicit education values, adapt one of three professional personae. Some of the threads mentioned by these authors are certainly evident in nursing students.

The student with a *technical persona* views being a good physician as the ability to perform technically. It appears that equating technical skill to good nursing is evident in students, especially early on in the program. Initially students focus on skills as what it means to be a nurse. The technical persona student, according to Coulehand and Williams, tends to be a skeptic and may develop a detachment from nonstudents, seeing the educational experience and faculty, nurses, or even patients as alienated from them. From anecdotal teaching experience in nursing programs, we believe that student alienation is also seen in nursing and that it can be observed as an individual response but also as a group phenomenon. Students who are alienated band together with others who are like-minded and who promote alienating and negating attitudes. Coulehan and Williams also believe that the technical persona student appears to be more detached from caring for their patients than other students, and may exhibit a heightened sense of entitlement.

A second persona is described as *nonreflective*. These individuals adopt behaviors from tacit learning and substitute intervention with personal interaction, are overly intense and often aggressive in their approach to treatment, and conflate self-interest with patient interest. These students may be too compliant, tend to be critical of patient care from others, and provide too many rather than too few interventions. Although not described by Coulehan and Williams, this second persona may relate to students who are unable to use phronesis in a fitting way.

The third group of students exhibits an *immune persona*. These students nourish an altruistic professional persona and have a "natural immunity" to the conflict of tacit and explicit curricula. Coulehan and Williams (2003) admitted that this type of student persona is poorly understood, but that a strong pre-professional personal commitment to social and religious ideals seems to be an antecedent factor. Older students and females, they claimed, may bring a greater "natural immunity" to the educational system conflict and complete the programs more successfully.

A second publication of interest was a study of the personalities of dental students to determine if personal traits impacted a student's success as a professional. First, the researchers compared students' personality profiles with actively practicing dentists and, second, students were evaluated to determine if their personal traits were useful predictors of success in the dental education (Chamberlain, Catano, & Cunningham, 2005). The researchers found that both positive and negative personal qualities like agreeableness, conscientiousness, anger, depression, and impulsiveness were predictive of success, but the more positive qualities were also significant when compared to practitioners. The successful students were more consistent with the personality profiles of the practitioners than were the less successful students. The researchers concluded that, in dental students, personal characteristics play a role in the success of students and should be considered in the dental school selection process.

Character Development Through Patterns of Behavior

Instruments that measure behavior generally measure either positive or negative behaviors. The instrumentation that measures negative/unprofessional behaviors and attitudes of unprofessional behavior were the more popular measures in the early development of professionalism and ethics measures (Rogers et al., 2001). Measures of professional attitudes toward a variety of unprofessional behaviors included, among others, cheating, deceiving, and measurement of bias (Lynch et al., 2004). More recently, a few studies in medicine were conducted to determine if students with poor attitudes and problem behavior were more likely to be disciplined for unprofessional behavior once they were professionals (Hickson, Pichert, Webb, & Gabbe, 2007; Van de Camp, Vernooij-Dassen, Grol, & Bottema, 2006). Two different medical student studies (Papadakis et al., 2005; Papadakis, Hodgson, Teherani, & Kohatsu, 2004) reported that disciplinary action among practicing physicians was strongly associated with unprofessional behavior in medical school.

Antecedent Factors

Predictors of performance over time have been of interest to researchers in medicine and can be considered at preprofessional education, education, and postprofessional education junctures. The relationship of cognitive performance and future success on NCLEX has been well documented, but development of professional attitudes, character, and morality has not.

Most research on antecedent concepts has been a result of the resurgence of interest in professional education in medicine. A relationship among antecedents as predictors for performance in medical school by Stern, Frohna, and Gruppen (2005) in a sample of 183 students did not find a clear antecedent predictor of future performance. The antecedents used represented a wide range of variables that included, among many others, volunteerism, type of degrees held by the candidate, and interview ratings.

School Performance and Professional Practice

Research regarding professional education and postprofessional education suggests a significant relationship between medical students performance or attitudes documented during school, and attitudes and disciplinary actions taken posteducation as practitioners. Ainsworth and Szauter (2006) discovered that common features were observed in problem students and in professionals who were disciplined. Generally, Ainsworth and Szauter (2006) found that students who were disciplined were unable to reflect on their shortcomings and, even if shortcomings were known, these students were less likely to change behaviors that were undesirable or unacceptable. Papadakis and colleagues (2005), in a large national study, reported that medical students who received disciplinary actions while in school were significantly more likely to be recipients of disciplinary actions of the state board regulators when in practice. It is apparent that even simple slips, like failure to turn in work on time, may predict poor performance in clinical rotations and in later professional settings (Stern et al., 2005).

One study compared attitudes and behaviors in practicing professionals. The purpose of the study was to measure the consistency between practicing physicians' attitudes and their self-reported practices (N = 1662). Campbell and colleagues (2007) reported that attitudes held by physicians sampled did not always conform to their self-reported behaviors.

The authors have found no research that was longitudinally conducted with nurses to evaluate the relationship between behaviors and attitudes in nursing school and further professional disciplinary actions in practice.

MEASUREMENT OF THE GLOBAL CONSTRUCT OF PROFESSIONALISM

Some researchers and scholars have attempted to develop a global measure of professionalism. Lynch et al. (2004) identified 22 different instruments that had been developed to measure what was classified as either "professionalism behavior" or "comprehensive environment" from five databases from 1982 to 2002 (that did not include specific nursing databases). The nursing literature on professionalism in nursing education indicates that professionalism is assessed through qualitative measures, like portfolios, personal reflection, critical incidents, and evaluations. Only one instrument had been developed for assessing professionalism—the Professionalism in Nursing Inventory (PNI)—and that instrument was designed for use in practicing nurse populations and generally measured accomplishments and behaviors (Adams & Miller, 2001; Miller, Adams, & Beck, 1993).

Instruments that have proposed a more comprehensive view and measure professionalism as a global concept measured two aspects: attributes and behaviors. Some studies concentrated on the validation of what comprises professionalism in specific disciplines and on conceptual development that will ultimately lead to development of better measurement methods (Chisholm, Cobb, Duke, McDuffle, & Kennedy, 2006; Siegler, 2000; Weber, 2006).

Jha, Berker, Duffy, and Roberts (2006) conducted a comprehensive literature review of studies assessing attitudes toward professionalism that included the Cumulative Index to Nursing and Allied Health Literature (CINAHL®) and six other databases from 1980 to 2006. The researchers reviewed 97 studies, of which, the majority were samples of medical students in the United States. Over half of the studies assessed attitudes, beliefs, and opinions of individuals sampled. Additionally, 15 of these studies were longitudinal and only 3 of the 15 indicated that there were attitudinal changes over time. Jha et al. (2006) concluded that theoretical frameworks were lacking on which to conceptualize professionalism, that few instruments to measure professionalism existed, and that the relationship between attitudes and future behaviors and practice was poorly researched.

A number of nonnursing behavioral instruments are reported in the medical and other health-related fields. Professionalism behavior measures obtain a broad representation and may include multiple evaluators, from the students themselves, patients, peers, faculty, mentors, or other healthcare providers. Chisholm and colleagues (2006) have a well-developed instrument to assess pharmacy students' behaviors, the Pharmacy Professionalism Instrument (PPI), that, through factor analysis, has six subscales identified: respect for others, honesty/integrity, excellence, altruism, duty, and accountability. Physical therapy literature indicates that similar activities for developing professional behavior norms are in progress for that profession (Wolff-Burke, 2005).

Two other instruments that measure professional behaviors that are reported in the medical literature are of particular interest. Although the Nurse Evaluation of Medical Housestaff (NEMH; Butterfield & Mazzaferri, 1991) tool was initially for nurses to evaluate resident doctors, the instrument is reported reliable and, according to Lynch et al. (2004), may be adopted for use with other evaluators.

A second instrument, the University of Michigan Department of Surgery Professionalism Assessment Instrument (UMDSPAI; Gauger, Gruppen, Minter, Colletti, & Stern, 2005), is the only instrument that we found that used a semantic differentiation format. The UMDSPAI is structured so that behaviors and character traits or virtues can be rated according to fit in the clinical setting. The student being evaluated could be observed doing a particular professional indicator or be perceived as having too little or too much of that indicator. The best score on the UMDSPAI was if students were rated with the median rating because it meant that the student evaluated was practicing in the most appropriate and fitting ways.

For example, the goal of "virtue" might be humility, which, on the UMDSPAI, will correspond to "response to criticism" and the scale ranks low and high scores. The lowest scores indicate the student has "immediate and vocal denial of issue, attempts to divert blame to others," indicating that the student has too little ability to use humility properly or in a balanced way. On the other side of too much humility, the students "takes criticism too much to heart. Takes a performance problem and personalizes it." This high score indicates that the student has used the virtue of humility too severely on himself or herself. The middle scores of the category "response to criticism" exhibits a reasoned response that is using the humility properly—"accepts criticism without personal offense. Uses criticism to improve performance visibly"— would represent proper use of phronesis and a balanced approach to using humility in practice and comportment. The UMDSPAI appears to measure behaviors that are general enough to be applicable to other disciplines, especially for disciplines that include clinical practice and evaluation. We believe that it is the best model for quantitative measure of professionalism that we have seen and one that explicitly evaluates a student's ability to balance and properly contextualize her practice.

DEVELOPING STRATEGIES FOR EVALUATING PROFESSIONALISM

Professionalism, when conceptualized in all its richness, and as seen in the previous chapters, is central to nursing and should be an explicit, intentional focus of curricula that is clearly used to shape nurses' practice and professional life. In curricula, professional development as a lifelong transformational process should be addressed early, repeatedly, and be integrated into classroom and clinical experiences and use a variety of already developed strategies (Table 7-2).

There are several general dimensions of professionalism that are critical to professional development if the FrNP and the Stairstep Model of Professional Transformation are used as the conceptual basis for professionalism curricula. Evaluation of student professional development will be sufficient only if both social and psychological elements of professionalism are addressed and if professionalism is approached as an aspirational and transformational process that can be evaluated over time. The measurement of professionalism, whether global or as parts of a construct, should be strengthened conceptually and psychometrically. It is evident from literature that further work is needed toward reliable and valid instrumentation that is based on a theory or framework. Too much standardization may stifle the creative ways of evaluation that that might emerge with a fuller conceptualization of professionalism, as with the FrNP. The diversity of nursing education programs best fits with allowing faculty the freedom to determine the best forms of educating and evaluating the nurse professional in their respective programs.

Based on the proposed framework and our literature review, we can offer guidance in methods that promote sufficient evaluation of professionalism in nursing curricula. Many nursing programs already incorporate some of the methods described herein.

Psychological Evaluation of Professionalism

A psychological evaluation of professionalism is essential and provides the evaluator with a glimpse of the inner world, virtues, character traits, and decision-making capacities of the student nurse. For psychological evaluation based on the FrNP, character can be measured by attitudes, values, personal professional ideals held, understanding and adherence to social constructs of professionalism, or social professional ideal.

Table 7-2   Potential Evaluators of Professionalism

Self	Instructor/mentor
Peer	Patient
Upper- and underclassmen	Other team members/providers

Psychological aspects are clearly the most challenging parameters to assess. One of the most significant problems with students' perceptions of themselves is their willingness to be honest and reflective in evaluating their ethical and professional development. Students often know what they "should" do opposed to what they "would really" do. The chasm between theory and practice can be wide and can make self-evaluation and measurement in areas that might impact their success as a student challenging.

There are a number of qualitative strategies that may improve evaluation of individual student progress, and that can be used in conjunction with other quantitative methods. The quantitative instruments presented previously are representative of the quantitative instruments available. Reflection as a method for psychological evaluation in general and then two specific methods that incorporate reflection are discussed.

Reflection

Student reflection can be used to educate or to evaluate and has not been fully utilized as such (Gustafsson & Fagerberg, 2004). Reflection and reflective practice have been considered from an epistemological perspective (Kinsella, 2007) as well as from a moral perspective. The difference between epistemology and ethical perspectives are summed up as *knowing what to do* (knowledge) and *knowing if one should do it* (ethics). Reflection of the professional is, as many experts in professional education claim, an ethical endeavor that leads to transformation (Kinsella, 2007). Reflection of practice represents one of the key elements of education and process evaluation when viewed through the FrNP.

Journaling and Critical Incidents

Students are often assigned to journal about clinical experiences and their personal responses. These reflections can be intentionally directed to facilitate student learning as well as inform the evaluator of student professional development. Critical incidents (CIs) methodology is a way of structuring reflection and is reported to assess professional traits of responsibility, reliability, self-assessment, respect, integrity, and maturity (Papadakis & Lõeser, 2006; Schluter, Seaton, & Chaboyer, 2008). A problem behavior is reported and evaluated longitudinally as patterns so that one incident is not too heavily weighted. Patterns emerge and further reports made so that remedial actions can be taken.

The original intent of CIs was for identification of individuals who are having problems rather than identifying and reinforcing good decisions and actions. One report of the use of a CI method is called *guided reflection* and is designed to prepare medical students for professional practice (Stark, Roberts, Newble, & Bax, 2006). A video of a doctor–patient, doctor–nurse, or nurse–patient encounter is shown and each student reflects individually and then discusses the response in a small group. CI methods provide prompts to help students work through a reflective process. Nursing educators are conscious of the value of positive reinforcement for students while in their educational experience. Reinforcement of positive actions is as important as constructive criticism because it helps our students to appreciate and develop a proclivity toward phronesis—to think and do similar good work in the future.

Portfolios

Portfolios also have both instructional and evaluative value for nursing education (Fryer-Edwards, Pinsky, & Robins, 2006; Karlowicz, 2000). A portfolio is a collection of achievements that attest to an individual's progress. The information in a portfolio can be varied and may contain videos or DVDs, pictures, narratives, awards, letters, or other items that showcase the individual student achievements and reinforces life-long learning and growth in the process of becoming a nurse professional. Kalet and colleagues (2007) reported using a unique Web-based program that requires regular entry of portfolio updates. Portfolios help to reinforce and maintain the portrait of the ideal professional self and to encourage aspiration toward it.

Portfolios, structured and unstructured reflection of clinical experiences, and critical incidents that are the qualitative measures of professionalism (as well as the more quantitative approaches like surveys that assess moral development or particular attitudes or perceptions) can be used to measure the psychological indicators of professional growth and transformation. Clearly additional work and research toward determining conceptual consistency of these methods for a given curriculum, the development of sufficient methods to evaluate, and the use of these methods properly are needed.

Interprofessional Perceptions

Interprofessional education (IPE) and collaborative practice, is not only an obvious strategy for the social aspects of professional education, but also has potential to be useful for evaluating psychological professional development. IPE has been shown to have a significant impact on attitudes toward other professionals and to also improve knowledge (MacKay, 2004). IPE of students can be useful in building their personal "professional portrait of the ideal" (Harris, 2008) by contrasting nursing students to other professionals and students from other disciplines. Students' awareness is raised of the similarities and differences among professions and in the common goals of health care.

Outcomes evaluation in IPE is an identified area of strength in IPE education (MacKay, 2004). Using a literature review, MacKay designed a strategy for evaluation of IPE by synthesizing two instruments, one of which is the nursing role Perception Questionnaire (Carpenter, 1995)—a reliable and valid instrument battery to measure student outcomes in other professions. MacKay named the instrument battery the role perception questionnaire. Seven factors emerged through factor analysis: breadth of professional outlook, degree of patient interaction, projected professional image, perception of personal professional status, possession of variety of skills, rapport with others, and degree of professional independence. The role perception questionnaire battery includes questions that address both the social and psychological domains of the individual student.

Quantitative Measures of Professional Growth

The quantitative measures of professional growth can be consistent with either social or psychological measures. In cases of quantitative measure, instruments have conceptual and metric limitations. The review of the instruments used for professionalism evaluation strongly suggested that further work toward developing reliable and valid instruments is necessary. There appears to be two fairly consistent general rules of thumb for quantitative measure: measure often and use a variety of sources. Measuring often is time intensive and requires more effort to develop an intentional plan for formative evaluation. Methods that establish growth by longitudinal study from assignment to assignment, from week to week, or from one semester or even one course to another are preferred. The evaluation of any student is looking for patterns of behavior rather than single incidences or "slips" in their progress toward the proper use of phronesis. A longitudinal array of evaluations will help to identify patterns rather than limit evaluation to single incidences. A variety of observers also increase the likelihood of valid evaluations.

In the review of instruments, we found that the UMDSPAI (Gauger et al., 2005) came closest to our conceptualization of professionalism as virtues or character traits by using a semantic differentiation scale. The UMDSPAI evaluated both virtues/character traits and behaviors for the traits, which appears to be unique to the instrumentation currently used in evaluation of professional development or ethics. Of course, this instrument, or one developed using this similar idea would be only part of a program developed to assess professional development in nursing education and/or practice. Table 7-3 includes two examples of what a semantic differentiation scale might look like for nursing. The ideal response is one that is balanced; the student knows how to use a virtue properly in a contextual setting. The better scores for this type of instrument would be a "3" or median.

Assessing a Professional Development Program

If professionalism and professional development were based on the FrNP and the virtue ethics tradition, the evaluation program will differ somewhat from traditional evaluative methods and would necessitate a greater degree of planning (Table 7-1). A helpful way to remember the general strategies for assessing professionalism is what we call the three Ms of professionalism: *multiple times*, *multiple people*, and *multiple methods*. In view of the previous review, the personal and professional ideal needs a greater degree of explicit identification and development across the curriculum. The personal professional ideal and the social professional ideal together becomes a clear portrait to which the student aspires in his or her professional development in school and in their professional life.

Table 7-3 Example Questions of Semantic Differentiation Used for Nursing Professional Development Evaluation

	1	2	3*	4	5
Compassion	Little interaction with patient other than directions, stays in room for minimal amount of time, must be asked to provide service rather than student anticipate needs	Superficial conversation with patient, limits going into patient care area, offers service in a general care way, anticipates some needs	Appropriate levels of deep or superficial communication used, stays in room for appropriate lengths of time, addresses needs specifically for the patient and anticipates needs, encourages self-help when appropriate	Inappropriate use of deep conversation for the situation, appears to be in room excessively, hovers over patient, anticipates needs and does for the patient what they can do and would prefer to do for themselves	Use of deep conversation that is disturbing or probing to the patient, remains in room such that patient asks the student to leave, obsequious attitude, does everything for the patient
Integrity	Denies the truth when confronted	Discloses partial truth or tells truth if it is likely to be discovered	Discloses the truth when discovered, reports to appropriate people	Volunteers truth when student discovers it and tells inappropriate people	Is paralyzed by discovering the truth, discusses inappropriately, and is unable to move beyond the issue

*most fitting answer

REFERENCES

Adams, D., & Miller, B. K. (2001). Professionalism in nursing behaviors of nurse practitioners. *Journal of Professional Nursing, 17*(4), 203–210.

Ainsworth, M. A., & Szauter, K. M. (2006). Medical student professionalism: are we measuring the right behaviors? A comparison of professional lapses by students and physicians. *Academic Medicine, 81*(10), 10S.

American Nurses Association. (1998). *Code of ethics for nurses.* Washington, DC: Author.

Arnold, L. (2002). Assessing professional behavior: yesterday, today and tomorrow. *Academy of Medicine, 77,* 502–515.

Association of American Colleges and Universities. (2010). *Cognitive-structural measurements of personal and social responsibility development in students.* Available online at http://www.aacu.org /core_commitments/CognitiveStructuralMeasurements.cfm. Accessed January 26, 2010.

Baldwin, D. C., & Self, D. J. (2006). The assessment of moral reasoning and professionalism in medical education. In D. T. Stern (Ed.), *Measuring medical professionalism* (pp. 75–93). New York: Oxford University Press.

Bebeau, M. J. (2002). The defining issues test and the four component model: Contributions to profession education. *Journal of Moral Education, 31*(3), 271–295.

Bebeau, M. J., Rest, J. R., & Yamoor, C. M. (1985). Measuring dental students' ethical sensitivity. *Journal of Dental Education, 49,* 225–235.

Braithwaite, V. A., & Law, H. G. (1985). Structure of human values: testing the adequacy of the Rokeach Value Survey. *Journal of Social Psychology, 49,* 250–263.

Butterfield, P. S., & Mazzaferri, E. L. (1991). A new rating form for use by nurses in assessing residents' humanistic behavior. *Journal of General Internal Medicine, 6,* 155–161.

Campbell, E. G., Regan, S., Gruen, R. L., Ferris, T. G., Rao, S. R., Cleary, P. D., et al. (2007). Professionalism in medicine: Results of a National Survey. *American College of Physicians, 147*(11), 795–802.

Carpenter, J. (1995). Interprofessional education for the medical and nursing students: Evaluation of a programme. *Medical Education, 29,* 265–277.

Chamberlain, T. C., Catano, V. M., & Cunningham, D. P. (2005). Personality as a predictor of professional behavior in dental school: comparisons with dental practitioners. *Journal of Dental Education, 69*(11), 1222–1237.

Chisholm, M. A., Cobb, H., Duke, L., McDuffle, C., & Kennedy, W. K. (2006). Development of an instrument to measure professionalism. *American Journal of Pharmaceutical Education, 70*(4), 1–6.

Coates, C. (1997). The caring efficacy scale: Nurses' self-reports of caring in practice settings. *Advanced Practice Nursing Quarterly, 3*(1), 53–59.

Colby, A., & Kohberg, L. (1987). *The measurement of moral judgment,* Volume 1. New York: Cambridge University Press.

Coulehan, J., & Williams, P. C. (2003). Conflicting professional values in medical education. *Cambridge Quarterly of Healthcare Ethics, 12,* 7–20.

Crigger, N. J. (1994). Universal prescriptivism: Traditional moral theory revisited. *Journal of Advanced Nursing, 20,* 538–543.

Davis, M. (2002). *Profession, code and ethics: toward a morally useful theory of today's professions.* Hants, UK: Ashgate Publishing Limited.

Dierckx de Casterlé, B., Izumi, S., Godfrey, N., & Denhaerynck, K. (2008). Nurses' response to ethical dilemmas in nursing practice: Meta-analysis. *Journal of Advanced Nursing, 63*(6), 540–549.

Duckett, L., Rowan, M., Ryden, M., Krichbaum, K., Miller, M., Wainwright, H., et al. (1997). Progress in the moral reasoning of baccalaureate nursing students between program entry and exit. *Nursing Research, 46*(4), 222–229.

Duckett, L., Rowan-Boyer, M., Ryden, M. D., Crisham, P., Savik, K., & Rest, J. R. (1992). Challenging the misperceptions about nurses' moral reasoning. *Nursing Research, 41*(6), 324–331.

Elman, N. S., Illfelder-Kaye, J., & Robiner, W. N. (2005). Professional development as a foundation for competent practice in psychology. *Professional Psychology, Research and Practice, 36*(4), 367–375.

Fleischmann, S. T. (2004). Essential ethics-embedding ethics into an engineering curriculum. *Science and Engineering Ethics, 10*, 369–381.

Fryer-Edwards, K., Pinsky, L. E., & Robins, L. (2006). The use of portfolios to assess professionalism. In D. T. Stern (Ed.), *Measuring medical professionalism* (pp. 213–234). New York: Oxford University Press.

Gastmans, C. (2006).The care perspective in healthcare ethics. In A. J. Davis, V. Tschudin, & L. La Raeve (Eds.), *Essentials of teaching and learning nursing ethics* (pp. 135–148). London: Churchill & Livingston.

Gauger, P. G., Gruppen, L. D., Minter, R. M., Colletti, L. M., & Stern, D. T. (2005). Initial use of a novel instrument to measure professionalism in surgical patients. *The American Journal of Surgery, 189*, 479–487.

Gilligan, C. (1982). *In a different voice: Psychological theory and women's development.* Cambridge, MA: Harvard University Press.

Gustafsson, C., & Fagerberg, I. (2004). Reflection, the way to professional development? *Journal of Clinical Nursing, 13*, 271–280.

Hare, R. M. (1989). *Moral thinking.* Oxford, UK: Clarendon Press.

Harris, C. E. (2008). The good engineer: Giving virtue its due in engineering ethics. *Science Engineering Ethics, 14*(2), 153–164.

Hickson, G. B., Pichert, J. W., Webb, L. E., & Gabbe, S. G. (2007). A complementary approach to promoting professionalism: identifying, measuring, and addressing unprofessional behavior. *Academic Medicine, 82*(11), 1040–1048.

Jha, V., Berker, H. L., Duffy, S. R. G., & Roberts, T. (2006). A systematic review of studies assessing and facilitating attitudes towards professionalism in medicine. *Medical Education, 41*, 822–829.

Kalet, A. L., Sanger, J., Chase, J., Keller, A., Schwartz, M. D., Fishman, M., et al. (2007). Promoting professionalism through an online professional development portfolio: successes, joys, and frustrations. *Academic Medicine, 82*(11), 1065–1072.

Karlowicz, K. A. (2000). The value of student portfolios to evaluate undergraduate nursing programs. *Nurse Educators, 25*(2), 82–87.

Kinsella, E. A. (2007). Embodied reflection and the epistemology of reflective practice. *Journal of Philosophy of Education, 41*(3), 395–409.

Kohlberg, L. (1981). *The philosophy of moral development stages and the idea of justice.* San Francisco: Harper & Row.

Kovach, R. A., Resch, D. S., & Verhuist, S. J. (2009). Peer assessment of professionalism: A five year experience in medical clerkship. *Journal of General Internal Medicine, 24*(6), 742–746.

Lemonidou, C., Papathanassoglou, E., Giannakopoulou, G., Patiraki, E., & Papadatou, D. (2004). Moral professional personhood: ethical reflections during initial clinical encounters in nursing education. *Nursing Ethics, 11*(2), 122–137.

Lynch, D. C., Surdyk, P. M., & Eiser, A. R. (2004). Assessing professionalism: A review of the literature. *Medical Teacher, 26*(4), 366–373.

MacKay, S. (2004). The role perception questionnaire (RPQ): A tool for assessing undergraduate students' perceptions of the role of other professionals. *Journal of Interprofessional Care, 18*(3), 289–302.

McAdams, D. P. (2009). The moral personality. In D. Narvaez & D. K. Lapsley (Eds.), *Personality, identity, and character: explorations in moral psychology* (pp. 11–29). New York: Cambridge University Press.

Miller, B. K., Adams, D., & Beck, L. (1993). A behavioral inventory for professionalism in nursing. *Journal of Professional Nursing, 9*(5), 290–295.

Myyry, L., & Helkama, K. (2002). The role of value priorities and professional ethics training in moral sensitivity. *Journal of Moral Education, 31*(1), 35–50.

Narvaez, D., & Lapsley, D. (2009). *Personality, identity and character: Explorations in moral psychology.* New York: Cambridge University Press.

Papadakis, M., & Loeser, H. (2006). Using critical incident reports and longitudinal observations to assess professionalism. In D. T. Stern (Ed.), *Measuring medical professionalism* (pp. 159–174). New York: Oxford University Press.

Papadakis, M. A., Hodgson, C. S., Teherani, A., & Kohatsu, N. D. (2004). Unprofessional behavior in medical school is associated with subsequent disciplinary action by a state medical board. *Academy of Medicine, 79,* 244–249.

Papadakis, M. A., Teherani, A., Barach, M. A., Knettler, T. R., Rattner, D. T., Stern, D. T., et al. (2005). Disciplinary action by medical boards and prior behavior in medical school. *The New England Journal of Medicine, 353,* 2673–2682.

Patenaude, J., Niyonsenga, T., & Fafard, D. (2003). Changes in students' moral development during medical school: A cohort study. *Canadian Medical Association Journal, 168*(7), 840–844.

Pellegrino, E. D. (2006). Toward a reconstruction of medical morality. *American Journal of Bioethics, 6*(2), 65–71.

Quiantance, J. L., Arnold, L., & Thompson, G. S. (2008). Development of an instrument to measure the climate of professionalism in a clinical teaching environment. *Academic Medicine, 83*(10), 55–58.

Rassin, M. (2008). Nurses' professional and personal values. *Nursing Ethics, 15*(5), 615–630.

Rest, J. R. (1986). *Moral development advances in research and theory.* New York: Praeger.

Rogers, G., Mentkowski, M., Hart, J. R., & Minik, K. S. (2001). *Disentangling related domains of moral, cognitive, and ego development.* Paper presented at American Educational Research Association, Seattle, Washington, April 2001.

Rokeach, M. (1973). *The nature of human values.* New York: Free Press.

Sadler, J. (2003). A pilot study to measure the caring efficacy of baccalaureate nursing students. *Nursing Education Perspectives, 24*(6), 295–299.

Schluter, J., Seaton, P., & Chaboyer, W. (2008). Critical incident technique: A user's guide for nurse researchers. *Journal of Advanced Nursing, 61*(1), 107–114.

Schwartz, S. (1992). Universals in the content and structure of values: theoretical advances and empirical tests in 20 countries. *Advances in Experimental Social Psychology, 25*, 1–65.

Siegler, M. (2000). Professional values in modern clinical practice. *Hastings Center Report, 30*(4), S29.

Stark, P., Roberts, C., Newble, D., & Bax, N. (2006). Discovering professionalism through guided reflection. *Medical Teacher, 28*(1), e25–e31.

Stern, D. T., Frohna, A. Z., & Gruppen, L. D. (2005). The prediction of professional behavior. *Medical Education, 39*, 75–82.

Swanson, K. (1999). What is known about caring in nursing science: A literature meta-analysis. In A. S. Hinshaw, S. Feetham, & J. Shaver (Eds.), *Handbook of clinical nursing research* (pp. 31–60). Thousand Oaks, CA: Sage.

Thorpe, K., & Loo, R. (2003). The values profile of nursing undergraduate students: Implications for education and practice. *Journal of Nursing Education, 42*(2), 201–204.

Van de Camp, K., Vernooij-Dassen, M., Grol, R., & Bottema, B. (2006). Professionalism in general practice: Development of an instrument to assess professional behavior in general practitioner trainees. *Medical Education, 40*, 43–50.

Veloski, J. J., Fields, S. K., Boex, J. R., & Blank, L. (2005). Measuring professionalism: A review of studies with instruments reported in the literature between 1982 and 2002. *Academic Medicine, 80*(4), 366–370.

Weber, J. A. (2006). Business ethics training: Insights from learning theory. *Journal of Business Ethics, 70*, 61–75.

Weis, D., & Schank, M. J. (2000). An instrument to measure professional nursing values. *Journal of Nurse Scholarship, 32*(2), 201–204.

Weis, D., & Schank, M. J. (2009). Development of psychometric evaluation of the Nurses Professional Value Scale–Revised. *Journal of Nursing Measurement, 17*(3), 221–231.

Wolff-Burke, M. (2005). Clinical instructors' descriptions of physical therapist student professional behaviors. *Journal of Physical Therapy Education, 19*(1), 67–76.

Yeun, E., Kwon, A., & Ahn, O. (2005). Development of a nursing professional values scale. *Taehan Kanho Hakhoe Chi, 35*(6), 1091–1100.

CHAPTER 8

Virtues Significant in Nursing

For the fruit of the Spirit is love, joy, peace, patience,
kindness, goodness, faithfulness, gentleness and self-control.

—GALATIANS 5:22 NIV

This above all: to thine own self be true, and it must follow,
as the night the day, thou canst not then be false to any man.

—WILLIAM SHAKESPEARE, *Hamlet*

Of the many rich contributions that have been passed down from Aristotle and through the virtue ethics tradition, none has been more widely accepted in moral dialogue than has the idea of virtues themselves (Mayo, 1985). Virtue has been in use for centuries to describe positive qualities of the psyche, and naturally fits with ordinary language and common sense beliefs. Someone with no knowledge of virtue ethics still understands and uses the word virtue.

Each of the individual virtues has a shared general understanding but becomes highly specific when the virtue is applied to individual life situations. Compare the function of virtues to gloves. A pair of gloves is standard size but the fiber or leather of which the gloves are made is designed to stretch to fit to the hands of the user. Once purchased and worn the gloves cleave to the hands, making the glove specific to fit the hand. Virtues are similar; they have common consensus but are contextually applied by individuals to particular situations.

In this chapter, the authors present a further discussion of virtues. The authors have selected four virtues that we believe to be fundamental to nursing and its practice: compassion, integrity, humility, and courage. Two of the selected virtues are strongly advocated as critical in our discipline. Compassion or caring, and integrity are well documented, ethically significant concepts in the nursing literature. Moral courage is addressed in nursing literature but to a lesser degree, and humility, although it has a long history as a moral concept, has only recently reemerged in the philosophical literature with a more contemporary conceptualization. Humility, if understood in a more contemporary frame, has the potential to add significantly to nursing professionalism. In each case, the virtue is conceptualized briefly with particular attention to its practical application in nursing.

VIRTUES AND FAITH ORIENTATIONS

The virtue ethics tradition is useful in professional education and specifically in the Framework for Nurse Professionals (FrNP) because of its compatibility with both faith-based and nonfaith-based orientations. Religious traditions of the ancient world, some of which predate classical Aristotelian thought, fall under the same rubric as virtue tradition. Like the classical virtue ethics tradition, prominent world religions emphasize character development and add the dimension of the supernatural as having an impact on the natural world and on human behavior. In some religious traditions, individual characteristics or virtues are the result of supernatural gifting or regeneration of the individual's spirit, while secular world views explain virtues as originating from a purely natural condition. People of faith may see virtue as a gift from God whereas others see their personal ethical development as their own achievement.

Whether from a religious or nonreligious perspective, individual character development is an important element of being human and is, in turn, fundamental to professionalism. From a pragmatic perspective, a difference in belief of the source of virtues or the ability to use them should not hinder recognition and development of the virtues themselves. In both cases, "good" is evident through exercising the virtue properly.

VIRTUES IN PRACTICE

Virtues, we have learned, are dispositions of character of an individual that, if used in a balanced and fitting way, result in flourishing for the individual moral agent, reinforcing using the virtue in a balanced way in the future, and achieving good outcomes. Aristotle categorized virtues as either *physical* or *moral* and defined four cardinal virtues: justice, temperance, prudence, and courage. Virtues vary in their qualities and may not work in the same ways. For example, integrity or prudence are portrayed as general or orientation virtues and act to ground other virtues, whereas other virtues, like courage, are more instrumental and result in action of the agent (Pellegrino & Thomasma, 1993; Sekerka & Bagozzi, 2007).

Aristotle, as well as many modern analyses of the virtue tradition, recognized that particular virtues were not universally valued (Jansen, 2000). There appears to be some virtues, like integrity, bravery, and love for family (philia), that might be valued universally, but any virtue may vary in value according to culture, society, institution, relations, and even the individual. Aristotle claimed that what counts as a virtue, although strongly influenced by society, is ultimately decided by the individual.

Student Nurses S and Y illustrate the individual nature of valuing virtues. Student Nurse S values knowledge as her professional ideal, so she aspires to acquire more knowledge in striving toward that ideal. Student Nurse Y's professional ideal of the nurse that she aspires to be is one who is compassionate. Each student must take an elective course. Can you guess which course might be chosen by each of the students? Student Nurse S selects a course on intermediate pharmacology and Student Nurse Y chooses to nurture her ideal through a course on communication and caring. From an external perspective, neither class should be preferred, unless our own personal professional ideal affects our perceptions of the situation. The nurse educator's role is to help students balance their personal professional portraits of the ideal nurse with their personal desires so that any one area of professional nursing and practice is not neglected.

Virtues have also been called *multi-track* (Hursthouse, 2009). Multi-track means that a person is not considered to be virtuous by a single act of using the virtue well. For example, Nurse R is able to act decisively and appropriately when she discovers that she has given a wrong medication. She discloses her mistake, apologizes to the appropriate people, and makes amends. The one incidence of honesty does not make her a person of integrity. Rather, virtues develop over time as a useful disposition that permeates every aspect of the individual and is evident in other actions, perceptions, attitudes, and one's ideals. A virtuous person is one who consistently uses the virtue properly.

As one is beginning to use virtues properly there is a tension between the right moral decision and action, and other less moral choices. The beginning stages of properly using virtues may be clouded by self-interests, carelessness, and the failure to act or "weakness of will" (Hare, 1991; Sekerka & Bagozzi, 2007). The right choices and actions create, over time, a pattern of using the virtue correctly, thereby creating a habit. A person is considered virtuous, when, according to most accounts, the virtue becomes second nature and the individual gives no serious consideration for deciding and acting in any other way than by proper use of the appropriate virtue. Proper exercise of virtues also promotes, transforms, and maintains the nurse professional's ideal of the good nurse, or what we have chosen to call the *professional ideal*.

Virtues are culturally and socially bound and often change over time. Looking back in history, the relationship of nurses with physicians has certainly changed over time and is illustrative of the fluidity of values. As a student in the late 1960s and early 1970s, deference toward physicans was valued. It was customary for nurses to offer the physician his or her seat if there were no available seats at the unit desk. It was also not unusual for a physician (almost exclusively male) to become verbally disrespectful to nurses. Little was done by administration or other healthcare providers when physicians were disrespectful unless the behavior was so blatant that it could not be ignored. Nurses were valued if they were patient, unquestioning, and followed physicians' orders.

Fortunately, unethical and disrespectful behaviors from any healthcare professional are no longer tolerated. The physician as the captain of the ship of previous years was replaced by a healthcare team with team members who are colleagues, who respect each other, and who work together for the best interests of the patient. Values of healthcare institutions have also changed and policies are in now place to ensure respect for all and to enact consequences for unethical behavior—replacing formerly unequal social healthcare cultural norms.

There are important differences in how each discipline views virtues. Professional disciplines or groups may value some virtues in their members more than they do others. The military values loyalty and obedience (Bowman, 2006), engineers add respect for nature and technical virtues (Harris, 2008), and authors in medicine claim compassion, trustworthiness, prudence, and respect for patient autonomy (Pellegrino & Thomasma, 1993; Siegler, 2000) as central to medical practice. There is no complete list of virtues at the social level, and virtues are continuing to be "discovered" like the respect for nature with engineering. With the renewed interest in virtue ethics, and as disciplines work toward clearer articulation of the essential virtues of their profession, identification of a comprehensive list of virtues becomes even less likely.

Although significant virtues have been clearly identified and others suggested, de Raeve (2006) claimed that virtues in nursing are "relatively unexplored territory" (p. 106). The discussion of priorities, or even what should or should not count as a virtue, are beyond the scope of this book, but we believe virtues to be central moral concepts to nursing and hope that a greater recognition of the importance of virtues will be part of ethics and professionalism in the future.

THE DEVELOPMENT OF A VIRTUOUS NURSE PROFESSIONAL

Virtues, by most accounts and certainly by Aristotle's, are both nurture and nature. Although virtues are largely developed, Aristotle claimed that people may have natural proclivities or tendencies to have a greater capacity for developing certain virtues. Children, for example, are born with individual character proclivities but these are not virtues, according to Aristotle, until the child learns to use them properly.

Virtues are developed and become easier to use properly with practice. Initially, when one becomes aware, an individual moral agent struggles with what choices to make and actions to take. Moral knowledge of principles, rules, attitudes, traditions, and other social and psychological facts all come into consideration. In addition to the cognitive and moral knowledge, emotional, character, value, and affective responses along with past experience also influence morally relevant decisions.

When a nursing student enters a nursing program, he or she not only brings the historical baggage from life to this time and place, but also begin to learn a new set of rules, expectations, and information. In short, students learn how to think and act like a nurse as they develop the ideals, adopt the professional values, and raise sensitivity to morally relevant situations. As we have claimed previously, how to use these new values and skills is not explicit, and students often rely on other students, mentors, and educators to somehow observe and assimilate the necessary skills to think and act like a nurse.

Students develop the professional values and virtues that are deemed more significant in nursing. One of the clearest virtues valued in nursing is integrity. Student nurses who plagiarize or are dishonest in clinical activities are generally reprimanded, warned, and, if behaviors continue, dismissed. To illustrate, turn to the case of Student V. Student V charted that she performed a certain procedure, when, in fact, the procedure was not done. The nursing instructor approaches Student V; once confronted the student recognized her short comings, is shamed, and is remorseful. Her professional ideal of what society expects of a nurse changes and the recognition that honesty is essential becomes clearer. Her personal professional ideal of what she wants to be as a nurse also changes, and honesty becomes a priority. Throughout the rest of Student V's education she has opportunities to be honest in the proper way. Gradually, she develops a pattern of using integrity as she shows in the professional role. Integrity permeates her thinking and how she relates to others, and she uses honesty in all her encounters; her consideration of doing something dishonest from fear or personal expediency gradually diminishes in its persuasive ability. By the time Student V graduates from nursing school, the virtue is so well developed that Student V no longer sees dishonest choices or behaviors as an alternative to being a person of integrity in any personal or professional situation.

Again, we stress, virtue tradition is about acquiring virtues through using them appropriately and in a balanced way, as in the case of Student V. Some critics claim that not all virtues are subject to overuse. Is there ever a time, the argument goes, that one has too much compassion? In situations of care or compassion, this virtue can cloud decisions made to provide the best care for patients. One of the best examples of too much compassion can be seen with providers who treat patients with substance abuse. The goal of the recovery model is for the patients, from within themselves, to develop self-regulation (Fardella, 2008). In these instances, helping may enable patients to continue to live in their disease. Recovery begins when enabling ends; a person faces the consequences, becomes self-aware, and seeks change.

Certainly the nurse, in situations like recovery from addiction, senses the affective response of compassion. The nurse professional has feelings of empathy and sympathy for the mother whose children have been taken by the state because of her neglect caused by drug use. At the same time, the best interests of the patient are served if the nurse restrains the response to the mother's perceived wants of getting her kids back and focuses on the patient's need for rehabilitation. The nurse expresses empathy for the mother's suffering and provides emotional support for her but does not enable her to continue drug abuse by interventions that do not allow her to suffer the consequences of her poor choices.

VIRTUES SIGNIFICANT IN NURSING

Compassion

Compassion has many associate words and is sometimes confused with empathy, pity, sympathy, and caring. Empathy refers to one's ability to feel with another and although one cannot presume to actually experience another's feelings, one can imagine what another may be experiencing. Sympathy is feeling badly about the situation of another, as with death of a loved one, or a colleague who is diagnosed with cancer. Compassion is a two-part concept. Generally compassion is described as *feeling* with another (empathy) and being moved to *respond*; to do something to help (Pellegrino &

Thomasma, 1993). No discussion of compassion in nursing is complete without consideration of the concept of caring or the care ethic. Caring has developed over the past decades as an ethical concept with a multiplicity of uses (de Raeve, 2006; Gastmans, 2006) but appears to contain some element of affective responsiveness to another. The clear distinction in the difference between *caring for* and *caring about* has been part of the nursing literature for some time. *Caring about* refers to the affective response that one has to the person for whom one cares. Students may not initially feel that they care about (have an affective response toward) patients but can care for (doing for) them. In other words, the student performs care activities for patients but may not have the internal sense of emotional responsiveness toward them.

Noddings' (1984) theory of care has been identified as the most developed of the caring theories and describes caring as a three part response (Crigger, 2001). Initially one attends to another, affectively feels with another, and then experiences the need to help the other. The three part response is awareness, personal emotional response, and action. Interestingly, Noddings described the two elements of compassion as two of the three parts of caring in her theory of care (Noddings, 1984).

Because virtues are multi-track and extend to all facets of character, thought, and action, if compassion is fully functioning in any given individual the evidence of this virtue extends to all relationships with others, including colleagues, family, and friends as well as patients. Although the self is as legitimate a recipient of caring as any other person (Engster, 2005), the virtue of compassion is social and is turned outward to others. Educators have struggled with whether or not *caring*—or, from our viewpoint, *compassion*—is teachable and, if so, how students be taught to care (Crigger, 2001; Pence, 1983). Often caring education is left to role-modeling; nursing students learns to add caring *about* to the caring *for* patients. The student may first adopt the behaviors observed in the role model: gentle touch of the patient's hands, being present, validating patient preferences, and affirming words. Then the doing becomes the being; the student begins to internalize *caring about* the patient in addition to *caring for* as part of their ideal of the good nurse. The movement of *caring for* to include *caring about* has been described as a secondary response that occurs concurrently during the course of *caring for* patients.

A qualitative descriptive study (Crigger, 2001) of student nurses suggested that certain situations, sensory stimulation, similarities, or the perception of patient suffering and need may stimulate students to engage emotionally with the patient and begin the process of *caring about* the patient while they *care for* them (Table 8-1). Likewise, barriers exist that inhibit students from developing *caring about* their patients. Students reported that the newness of the situation reduced their ability to care about patients. Students explained that they are busy learning how to *care for* the patient—give medications, know the medicine, and organize their time—that they were less likely to care about the patient. If students were given additional clinical periods with patients, the students reported that they had a greater opportunity for developing an affective

Table 8-1   Factors That Stimulate Student Nurses' Affective Responsiveness to Patients

<u>Sensory Triggers</u>	Reciprocation
Patients' eyes	Statements of appreciation
Physical appearance	Calling student by name
Patient's voice	
	<u>Emotional Reactions</u>
<u>Patient Situations</u>	Surprise
Patient suffering and need	Fear
Patient being alone	Helplessness
Age	Sadness
<u>Similarities</u>	
Remind student of their relatives or	
someone they knew	
Had had similar life experiences	

Adapted from Crigger, N. (2001). Antecedents to engrossment in Nodding's theory of care. *Journal of Advanced Nursing, 35*(4), 616–623.

caring relationship or bond with the patient. Likewise, if the student did not perceive a patient need or if the family members were present, caring about occurred less frequently according to the sampled student participants.

The study suggests that student nurses' ability to develop *caring about* the patient is fragile, and can be hindered by circumstances. The individual student, having knowledge of caring or compassion, differs from learning *how* to develop the caring sense about the patient and *how* to make that *caring about* evident to others.

According to Noddings' (1984) theory, one learns *how* to care through first receiving care as a baby, child, and then as an adult from one's own family or a surrogate. The belief that one is nurtured to become a compassionate person is consistent with virtue tradition. If caring is taught then there may be a great deal to teach students and nurses not only to know that compassion is important and valued but also—and perhaps most importantly—to know *how* to care about the patient through proper use of compassion.

If compassion is learned as a child from family or care takers, then many of those lessons may go unlearned by students that we are teaching today. Students who are from dysfunctional family situations may have less developed compassion and less ability to demonstrate it to others because of their life situations and experiences. Demonstration of caring may also be culture bound and vary. Diminished development of compassion add to the burden of teaching not only what caring or compassion is but also how to demonstrate compassion in appropriate ways.

Is care consistent with compassion? Although a thorough comparison of the essential nature of care and of compassion is beyond our scope, one can see that there is a question of semantics and substance with the two words. There are at least two reasons why using the word compassion to describe nurse professionals practice may be preferred to using the word caring. Caring at present is still in need of development and cannot stand as a full moral concept (Engster, 2005; Jaworska, 2007), whereas compassion entails a fuller conceptualization as an ethical concept and has a more vibrant historical tradition. Second, compassion and caring both have an affective element but compassion also entails action. The person with compassion is moved to act on behalf of the other. The FrNP is to be inclusive of either term in referring to a central virtue for nursing rather than a developed theory or stand alone moral concept.

Humility

In the last two decades, there has been a resurgence of interest the word humility mainly by philosophers—in conjunction with the rise of virtue ethics—and, strangely enough, in the theoretical work done in mistakes theory (Andre, 2000).

A review of nursing literature over the last decade retrieved only one article on humility by de Vries (2004), who likewise had conducted a literature review in which no publications on humility were found in nursing literature. De Vries's (2004) view of humility was consistent with its meaning as a self-deprecating concept. Humility originally referred to humus or soil that, when applied to people, indicated a lowly state. In Jewish and Middle Eastern traditions, foot washing was generally done by slaves as one entered the home. The Christ-like behavior of washing of the feet of others, for example, is described as an act of humility and was a useful strategy, according to de Vries (2004), to teach reflection and self-growth.

The definition of humility has expanded from self-effacement into a broader psychological orientation that connects with other virtues and is strongly self-reflective. Humility is now generally understood as a disposition or virtue that enables one to assess one's self realistically (self-reflection) and to maintain one's self in esteem (self-love; Andre, 2000; Snow, 1995). The element of self-reflection has been of great interest and is now appearing in the literature as a strain of new terminology like "cultural humility" (Miller, 2009) and "diagnostic humility" (Lockwood, 2009).

There is much to say theoretically about the concept, but the focus of our work is to describe humility so that its value for nursing or any profession is evident. There is a clear cross-discipline consensus that humility is a common response to one's perception that one has done something wrong (Andre, 2000; Garcia, 2006). Humility also comes into play when one receives an honor or from personal accomplishments that can result in pride (Kupfer, 2003; Snow, 1995). In both cases humility orients the individual to have a *realistic view of self*. In the first case, shame results when one does not meet the expectation or ideal of what one should be; in the second case, one often has a sense of exhilaration at an accomplishment because of a perceived success. In both cases, the key appears to be the ability for restraint; one does not overreact to the psychological impact of failure or success.

In the case of failure, humility is used properly when the individual turns compassion inward toward the self and views the event as failure, reflects realistically on the situation, discloses the error to one's self and appropriate others, and makes amends when possible. One of the most significant aspects of humility with errors or perceived shortcomings is that these experiences can be used as catalysts for growth and change (Crigger, 2004; Martin, 1999). In instances of success, proper use of humility helps the individual view the success or accomplishment realistically and in a way that does not exaggerate self-importance. Humility is diminishing the likelihood that one will be arrogant, be closed to others' suggestions, and have an exaggerated sense of pride. Humility also affects others because, by seeing ourselves in a realistic and balanced way, we see others in that way as well. Humility shapes our world to be realistic. We see people and ourselves in rightful place with a higher power and/or in a rightful place in the universe (Garcia, 2006; Kupfer, 2003).

Humility is like a buoy that rides the waves of disappointments and accomplishments (Fig. 8-1). Waves are the accomplishments and bring personal highs that

Figure 8-1   Humility.

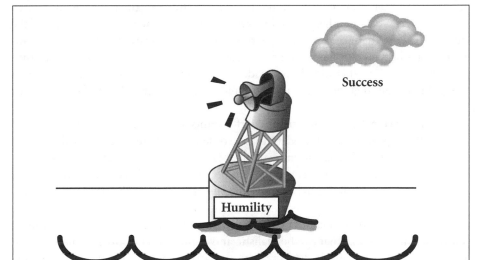

empower and build self-esteem, whereas the troughs of waves are the failures and dis-appointments that lower the sense of self-value and may result in shame or regret. In both cases, the buoy remains afloat on the ocean surface despite rough waters. Like the buoy, humility is a centering that keeps us either from extremes of losing anchor in the ocean and becoming airborne by the pride of self-achievement or from submerging in the ocean depths because of despair at our own weakness. If flying or sinking occurs, we have not held tightly enough to the buoy of humility and have disconnected with the realistic perspective of who and what we are.

Humility is highly significant for education and for personal and professional growth in general. Having the trait of humility that is developed well becomes an instrument to transform individuals for the better and helps them aspire to the ideal.

On one hand, riding the wave through positive experiences reinforces the individual to be successful. However, this success is not useful for students if they perceive success in an unbalanced way. Perfectionism and the desire to win may become too great and students become so intent on grades or winning that negative consequences occur. "Better is the enemy of good," (Voltaire, n.d.). Just this last semester, a nursing student who took one of the author's healthcare ethics courses emailed after receiving her grade. "I see," she wrote, "that I made a B+ on my final grade but I deserve an A." Certainly students should be concerned about grades and assertive with their concerns; however, the drive to succeed or win needs to be used in a balanced way. Students who place too great a value on success may also have a heightened sense of failure and, instead of riding the waves, are crushed by personal weaknesses and failures. Another student, also taking the same healthcare ethics course, illustrated the negative effects of a heightened reaction to failure. She approached one of the authors early in the semester, having earned a B on an essay exam. The student complained about the grade and began to cry openly. She was, she said, just not like this; she was better than this and always made A's on her work. Is her sense of failure so skewed that a good grade results in emotional pain? Can her feelings of self-worth be so fragile?

A difference between what student performance is and the personal ideal of what she should be producing was evident to the student. Some students rationalize or use other psychological defenses to mitigate their failures. However, excessive use of psychological defenses diminishes personal responsibility and becomes a barrier to an opportunity for growth. Denial of responsibility also removes the need for acknowledging a failure, seeking forgiveness, and making proper amends.

Humility, if understood and used in a fitting way, balances and explains errors or shortcomings in a way that can be realistic and helpful. If educators frame errors or weaknesses, as many already do, as realistically correctable shortcomings, the opportunities for growth from these experiences are possible. The proper use of virtues becomes evident only if errors and corrections can be made. Teaching students *how* to react ethically to errors and weaknesses that have resulted in problems are also important for students to learn. Humility, as one author claims, is "an attitude that is essential to clarity about oneself and to living with imperfection while striving mightily for something better" (Andre, 2000, p. 59).

Teaching students that they are vulnerable to errors and what to do when errors occur would be akin to the emergency plans that are recited before every airplane flight, or the practice of mustering to one's designated station when one is on a cruise ship. The public is taught what to do and how to do it if something goes wrong in the air or at sea. Errors in professional behavior should be handled in the same way. Certainly neither the educator nor the student intends to fail or make errors, but fallibility is an undeniable characteristic of being human. Mistakes are human beings being human. The likelihood that the nurse professional will make an error is far greater than an airplane crashing or a ship sinking. Yet, educators emphasize prevention of error and often ignore dealing proactively in preparing students to know how to respond to mistakes and shortcomings (Crigger, 2004).

Fowers and Davidov (2006) claim that multiculturalism is a virtue and that it is inclusive of the concept of cultural competence and respect for others. The authors (Fowers & Davidov, 2006) call the virtue of multiculturalism a moral imperative, that, when merged with virtue ethics, becomes the virtue of multiculturalism. Humility, by comparison, is more inclusive and assumes a broader view of respect for others than does multiculturalism. There is no logical reason that people from other cultures deserve more respect than any other person, as each human being should be given the same moral value as any other human being. Rather one looks to *how to* demonstrate respect and maintain dignity. Humility, in the more contemporary conceptualization, afford dignity and respect that is suggested by Fowers and Davidov (2006) for all people, including people of other cultures as well as people of one's own culture.

Some disciplines have identified virtues of particular significance to their members. Harris (2008), for example, has identified respect for nature as a contemporary virtue within the discipline of engineering. He describes two aspects of respect for nature: *perception of beauty* and *wonderment or awe*. This wonderment may also be akin to reverence toward nature in that there is a desire to keep it pristine, uncorrupted, and retained for the benefit of generations to come. Respect for nature then has two justifications: the intrinsic value of maintaining nature for its own sake but also the extrinsic value that maintaining nature has for human enrichment now and for future generations. Possessing the virtue of humility opens the individual to understanding that specific virtues might be part of other disciplines, and how they might be acted upon differently.

What can be concluded about humility in nursing? First, that its contemporary understanding is one of broadening humility into a moral virtue that orientates a person to the world and all things in it. The current understanding of humility incorporates forgiveness, respect for others, openness to others, and the use of compassion for the self. The nurse professional sees him or herself reflectively, realistically, and is able to ride the waves of success and failure, using either circumstance as transformational.

Integrity

Integrity, unlike humility, has been well identified in the professional literature and is considered a fundamental character trait or virtue. Integrity is strongly associated with honesty and truth telling (Hodkinson, 2008). Whereas humility deals with a person's orientation in relation to others and the universe, integrity deals with the relationship of the individual's inner connectedness and consistency with one's self. Personal integrity requires harmony and balance in order to maintain and honor commitments that one has made (Martin & Gabard, 2001; Prichard, 2006). Through balancing and honoring commitments, one is in harmony with what one thinks, speaks, and how one acts (Fig. 8-2). Integrity is exemplified by promise keeping, truth telling, and honesty. An individual is also authentic or sincere and does not resent or begrudge any of the commitments (Martin & Gabard, 2001).

Pellegrino and Thomasma (1993) viewed integrity as a fundamental virtue that is evident when the behavior of an individual is predictable. The case of Nurse C illustrates the predictable nature of a person of integrity. Nurse C has the reputation of being an expert nurse and has worked on the general surgical unit for 5 years. His supervisor knows this, and also knows from experience of working with him that Nurse C is a person of integrity. The supervisor trusts Nurse C and monitors Nurse C's practice minimally because of Nurse C's past performance and character. The supervisor trusts in Nurse C to do what is needed on the unit.

Figure 8-2   Integrity.

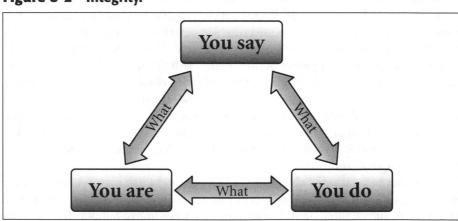

Integrity as a virtue is certainly important to the nurse professional but has its greatest impact on others and on their ability to trust. When patients trust their nurses they implicitly believe that that the nurse is their advocate and that nurses will act based on their best interests. Trust can be easily lost and is clearly important in the professional healthcare provider relationship (Crigger, 2009).

Courage

Courage, one of the classical cardinal virtues, has traditionally been categorized as either physical or moral. Physical courage is that which is done to protect or overcome physical harm, whereas moral courage deals with one's ethical commitments and integrity (Lachman, 2007). Putman (1997) claims that there is a third type of courage: psychological courage that relates to personal intemperance, like addictions or bad habits.

Some words conceptually overlap with courage. Fortitude is a type of sustained courage (Pellegrino & Thomasma, 1993). The idea of strength is made clearer if we consider the use of the stem word of *fortification*. As forts are buildings that offer protection and fortified milk is strengthened with vitamins or minerals, fortitude is the strengthening of the resolve of the individual to continue to be courageous. Bravery describes a quality of acts rather than a character disposition—although the word is sometimes used interchangeably with courage. Aristotle claimed that courage was motivated by nobility (one's good upbringing), success, victory, or because of the personal satisfaction that one would gain by being courageous.

Courage in professionalism is described as having two significant uses: to promote change, or to stand in opposition for moral rightness. In the first sense, in the professions, change is challenging and courage is a quality that is particularly desired in leaders (Lachman, 2007). Leaders have the moral courage and fortitude to continue holding to a vision of change and help direct others toward it despite risk and resistance (Purtilo, 2000). Leaders can also hold fast to certain beliefs despite societal consensus that change needs to occur.

Moral courage is the readiness to risk being harmed to uphold something of great moral value (Purtilo, 2000). Harm could be physical and include loss of finances, social standing, or any other threat perceived by the individual who will act with courage. From a broader perspective, courage is commitment because there is something at stake that can be lost and the individual chooses to act voluntarily (Purtilo, 2000). Moving to say what you believe and to further act on it are the signs of moral courage. Moral courage is instrumental in being able to use other virtues like integrity. In Figure 8-2, integrity is presented so that there is implied consistency among the three terms: thinking, saying, and doing. However, courage is the strength to follow through with thinking and to venture into the social realm of saying and doing (Fig. 8-3). Spence and Smythe (2007) discussed the psychological impact of manifesting courage as causing a dual sense of confidence and fear. On one hand the courageous individual

Figure 8-3   Courage.

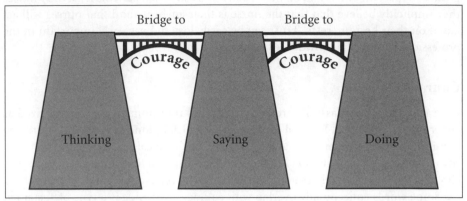

has a sense of confidence by believing that he or she is saying or doing the right thing and living up to the personal ideal, whereas on the other hand has the fear of suffering rejection or loss because of the courageous behavior.

Awareness of moral courage is limited and its significance in society may be underestimated (Purtilo, 2000; Sekerka & Bagozzi, 2007; Spence & Smythe, 2007). One misconception about moral courage is that, in human endeavors, moral courage is rare and extraordinary. In fact, being courageous enough to act on behalf of moral commitments and change should be, according to Sekerka and Bagozzi (2007), the expected norm for each professional.

In each case, the fear or danger that requires courage to overcome is real though the object of the fear may vary. In education, the question arises: Is moral courage teachable? Nursing educators highly value and teach students to value advocacy for their patients, but, are students instructed on what it takes to be an advocate and how to be one? Can students be taught that courage is much broader than saving a drowning child or saying no to cheating on exams? Courage can often describe everyday events. Students act bravely by being part of the clinical experience, and nursing instructors act bravely by confronting a student about a behavior in the clinical setting.

Suggestions for activating moral courage include helping students identify moral courage examples, and facilitating learning as students develop their personal professional ideal to include courage. It is important to teach students about how to use courage to make changes in their world, not just to teach about particular elements that are currently valued like multiculturalism, justice, leadership, or advocacy (Purtilo, 2000). Using imagination and role playing and attending to role modeling, especially with administration and leadership, can be helpful as well (Purtilo, 2000).

Lachman (2007) has developed a useful acronym for moral courage: CODE. C stands for courage, O for obligation to something for which the agent must be courageous about, D is for the danger of fear that is perceived, and E is to express the action. Lachman (2007) suggests that the individual who needs to mobilize courage should use a self-soothing approach, and reframe the situation. Self-soothing occurs when we use effective and strategic self-talk; imagination can be used to reframe intimidating situations or people or to encourage the fearful person to consider why it is important to take a stand. As a college student, one author remembers a suggestion to reduce fear of speaking was to find a friendly face in the audience and speak to that person. Lachman's (2007) suggestions are practical ways to improve the use of courage so that one follows through with words and actions.

CONCLUSION

Although ambiguity exists about virtues in a general sense, these virtues, as conceptualized through the virtue ethics tradition and through the FrNP, have practical significance for nursing education and practice. The authors have identified four fundamental virtues for nursing: compassion, integrity, humility, and courage. Together, these virtues communicate what is essential for the development of the personal professional ideal and are necessary to promote excellence in practice.

REFERENCES

Andre, J. (2000). Humility reconsidered. In S. B. Rubin & L. Zoloth (Eds.), *Margin of error* (pp. 59–72). Hagerstown, MD: University Publishing Group.

Bowman, J. (2006). *Honor: A history*. New York: Encounter Books.

Crigger, N. (2001). A qualitative study of the antecedents, to engrossment in Noddings' theory of care. *Journal of Advanced Nursing, 35*(4), 616–623.

Crigger, N. (2004). Always having to say you're sorry: An ethical response to making mistakes in professional practice. *Nursing Ethics, 11*(6), 568–576.

Crigger, N. J. (2009). Toward understanding the nature of conflict of interest and its application to the discipline of nursing. *Nursing Philosophy, 10*, 253–262.

de Raeve, L. (2006). A critique of virtue ethics. In A. J. Davis, V. Tschudin, & L. de Raeve (Eds.), *Essentials of teaching and learning in nursing ethics* (pp. 109–122). Edinburgh, UK: Churchill Livingston Elsevier.

de Vries, K. (2004). Humility and its practice in nursing. *Nursing Ethics, 11*(6), 577–587.

Engster, D. (2005). Rethinking care theory: The practice of caring and the obligation to care. *Hypatia, 20*(3), 50–74.

Fardella, J. A. (2008). The recovery model: Discourse ethics and the retrieval of the self. *Journal of Medical Humanities, 29*, 111–126.

Fowers, B. J., & Davidov, B. J. (2006). The virtue of multiculturalism: Personal transformation, character, and openness to the other. *American Psychologist, 61*(6), 581–594.

Garcia, J. L. A. (2006). Being unimpressed with ourselves: Reconceiving humility. *Philosophia, 34,* 417–435.

Gastmans, C. (2006). The care perspective in healthcare ethics. In A. J. Davis, V. Tschudin, & L. de Raeve (Eds.), *Essentials of teaching and learning nursing ethics* (pp. 135–148). Edinburgh, UK: Churchill Livingston Elsevier.

Hare, R. M. (1991). *Moral thinking: Its levels, method, and point.* Oxford, UK: Clarendon Press.

Harris, C. E. (2008). The good engineer: Giving virtue its due in engineering ethics. *Science and Engineering Ethics, 14,* 153–164.

Hodkinson, K. (2008). How should a nurse approach truth-telling? A virtue ethics perspective. *Nursing Philosophy, 9,* 248–256.

Hursthouse, R. (2009). Virtue Ethics. In E. N. Zalta (Ed.), *The Stanford encyclopedia of philosophy.* Available online at: http://plato.stanford.edu/archives/spr2009/entries /ethics-virtue.

Jansen, L. A. (2000). The virtues in their place: virtue ethics in medicine. *Theoretical Medicine, 21,* 261–276.

Jaworska, A. (2007). Caring and full moral standing. *Ethics, 117,* 460–497.

Kupfer, J. (2003). The moral perspective of humility. *Pacific Philosophical Quarterly, 84,* 249–269.

Lachman, V. D. (2007). Moral courage: A virtue in need of development? *MEDSURG Nursing, 16*(2), 131–133.

Lockwood, C. J. (2009). We need more diagnostic humility. *Contemporary OBGYN,* 12–13.

Martin, M. (1999). Explaining wrongdoing in professions. *Journal of Social Philosophy, 30*(2), 236–250.

Martin, M. W., & Gabard, D. L. (2001). Conflict of interest and physical therapy. In M. Davis & A. Stark (Eds.), *Conflict of interest in the professions* (pp. 314–332). New York: Oxford University Press.

Mayo, B. (1985). Virtue or duty? In C. H. Sommers & R. J. Fogelin (Eds.), *Virtue and vice in everyday life* (pp. 171–177). San Diego, CA: Harcourt Brace Jovanovich, Inc.

Miller, S. (2009). Cultural humility is the first step to becoming global care providers. *JOGNN, 38*(1), 92–93.

Noddings, N. (1984). *Caring: A feminine approach to ethics and moral education.* Los Angeles: University of California Press.

Pellegrino, E. D., & Thomasma, D.C. (1993). *The virtues in medical practice.* New York: Oxford University Press.

Pence, G. E. (1983). Can compassion be taught? *Journal of Medical Ethics, 9,* 189–191.

Prichard, M. S. (2006). *Professional integrity: Think ethically* [Monograph]. University of Kansas, Lawrence, KS.

Purtillo, R. B. (2000). Moral courage in times of change: Visions for the future. *Journal of Physical Therapy Education, 14*(3), 4–6.

Putman, D. (1997). Psychological courage. *Philosophy, Psychiatry, & Psychology, 4*(1), 1–11.

Sekerka, L. E., & Bagozzi, R. P. (2007). Moral courage in the workplace: moving to and from the desire and decision to act. *Business Ethics: A European Review, 16*(2), 132–149.

Siegler, M. (2000). Professional values in modern clinical practice. *Hastings Center Report, 30*(4), 4.

Snow, N. E. (1995). Humility. *The Journal of Value Inquiry, 29*, 203–216.

Spence, D., & Smythe, L. (2007). Courage as integral to advancing nursing practice. *Nursing Praxis in New Zealand, 23*(2), 43–55.

Voltaire. (n.d.). *BrainyQuote.com.* Available at: http://www.brainyquote.com/quotes/quotes/v/voltaire109643.html. Accessed June 12, 2010.

CHAPTER 9

Equipping the Next Generations of Nurse Professionals

If a calling is a moral life, then a professional calling cannot take root,
grow and flourish without a steady diet of ethics.

—SYLVESTER, 2002

The primary goal of any profession is to educate their members to be good professionals. The purpose of this book is to provide a thorough inquiry into the meaning and nature of professionalism, to learn from the wider landscape of ethics and other disciplines, and, through the knowledge gained, move nursing education forward so that nurses in future generations graduate as nurse professionals who are committed a life of professional growth. The final chapter is an exploration of what future trends might shape nursing professional education. In a way these trends are also ideals of how educators, as members of our profession, make themselves grow as they help in the making of nurse professionals.

EMERGING TRENDS IN NURSING

Two obvious truths will be evident in our profession's future: change and growing complexity of practice (Benner, Sutphen, Leonard-Kahn, & Day, 2010). At the macro level, change in the United States will be tied to the work done to make health care sustainable for the future. Nursing is in the process of expanding legitimate practice to include care that was formerly the exclusive practice of other professions. The profession is shifting to change education to meet the changes in practice and will be helping to shape the future of nursing education. There appear to be trends from many directions that will shape the future and the making of nurse professionals.

Trend #1: Fit, not Identity

Nursing is a young discipline and underdeveloped when compared to medicine, philosophy, or religion. The initial struggle in the discipline was one of identity. The discipline fought for distinction through unique diagnostic language, a specialized body of knowledge, and ethics particular to nursing. Predictions for now and the future are that nursing as a profession and a discipline will need to shift from one that is distinct from other disciplines to being focused on alignment with the healthcare system, on "advancing the goodness of fit between the external environment and the demand for continuous relevance in the internal environment" (Porter-O'Grady & Malloch, 2009, p. 247).

In today's world, the work of nursing should be about *fit* instead of *identity*. No longer is nursing trying to find its footing within the complex healthcare landscape or fighting for legitimacy as a profession. However, because of the speed at which global change occurs, the profession will need to quickly move away from irrelevance and fervently embrace the idea of *goodness of fit* as a central criterion for planning and action, because nursing is by no means as isolated as the discipline may have envisioned itself for the last five decades. Such a change will be a dramatic step, and will require a mindfulness and understanding about other disciplines, professions, and society. This level of engagement with other disciplines has historically been only partially embraced. Solutions to the complexity of health care and to societal problems now and in the future require that the discipline view itself with a greater degree of integration.

Trend #2: Value, not Volume

In nursing education, the questions will no longer be, "have we covered the content?" or "how much can they learn?" Instead, the questions become: "What difference is made by teaching ____?" "What is the impact of teaching these concepts in this way?" "Tell me what difference you're making." The need for education to be uncluttered has been evident to many educators for some time (Giddens & Brady, 2007). In a way, content-based teaching is like using crutches. It is much easier to teach content and test for it than tackle the more difficult areas or to change teaching styles. It is time to drop the crutches we use because we think volume is most important and, instead, do what will make an impact, or what will make a difference. Such a paradigm shift has the power to completely change the format for nursing education. Fortunately, a number of nurse educators and nurse leaders are already fostering this shift in thinking (Giddens & Brady, 2007; Ross, Noone, Luce, & Sideras, 2009; Vacek, 2009).

Trend #3: Are We Doing the Right Things, or Just Doing Things Right?

Nurses and nurse educators can become distracted by details that are not important to the final outcome. There are two reasons. First, nursing knowledge work is often detail work, so nurses have familiarity with such an approach. Second, in times of stress, it may be more self-regulating to "dig into the details." Problems arise when these details are actually workarounds and can ultimately be as counterproductive to unit goals. Covey's (1994) question, "Are we doing things right, or doing the right things?" illustrates how easily one can gravitate to minutia when that course of action is a poor choice. Consider the case of Nurse N, who spends 25 minutes teaching her hospitalized client who is ready for discharge about a low salt diet for his newly diagnosed hypertension. Such a nursing action would give the nurse manager cause for alarm: low salt diets are not effective for everyone and, in those for whom it works, the drop in blood pressure is usually approximately 1–3 mm Hg. This nurse's need to be thorough was an inappropriate action; the nurse was doing things right (perhaps meeting the nurse's own needs), but not doing the right things.

Trend #4: Put the Discipline of Nursing in the Center

Because of the landmark 2001 Institute of Medicine (IOM) report, *Crossing the Quality Chasm*, much of the conversation in health care is about patient-centered care. Patient-centered care fits well in a practice model; nursing practice has always been about service to the patient, the recipient of care. Said another way, practicing nurses have always viewed the patient at the "center of the circle." However, that practice model does not work as an educational model. If educators parallel the practice model and see graduation of the student as our primary concern then educators have abandoned their primary obligation as the gatekeepers of the discipline and to educate students who are nurse professionals prepared to take their places as members of our discipline. Instead, the authors contend that the discipline is in the center, because the educator's chief responsibility is to the discipline, in sufficiently preparing students to become *nurse professionals*, to become contributing members of the profession of nursing, and to serve society.

Professional education and our gatekeeper function have become more difficult in the face of social expectations. Consumerism and contemporary societal norms have influenced the development of an overly individualistic approach to nursing education. The university has become a business and the students have become consumers who feel entitled to receive the education. The desire and expectation to have students who receive training as an individualistic tailoring by the educator to meet their needs likely impairs the development of students' responsibility for their learning. Further, most professional programs cannot be designed to provide student-centered care at the level of patient-centered care in the hospital. Educational theory also suggested that catering to an individualistic approach may be detrimental to learning. Lave and Wenger's (1991) concept of *situated learning* as a central theme in professional education presumes that their term, "legitimate peripheral participation," is the norm for learning a profession because of the collective nature of a profession. In this model, the focus deliberately turns from the individual learner's needs and wants to reinforcing that each member learns from his/her membership in the group. As a result, that member becomes part of the profession. If the converse continues, and students are pedantically 'fed' facts and content without a well-developed professionalism context, they will increasingly demand that their education be delivered "as they want it," falsely giving legitimacy to a defeating cycle of higher education consumerism. Educating students for a top-tier profession cannot be done effectively using the same methods used in secondary settings or prerequisite college courses, or as learning is acquired in courses of study that do not lead to a profession. Further, professionalism cannot be taught using a market model driven by consumerism. The perspective is entirely different for professions. It is up to nursing education professionals to recognize this difference and clearly communicate it with students.

Trend #5: Move Students to a Critical–Systemic Way of Thinking

In Chapter 6 the authors addressed Parks's (1993) findings regarding students entering Harvard Business School. These students were expected to have moved to a *critical–systemic* way of thinking—yet, instead, they had stayed within their conventional ethos and were still at a *reflective–interpersonal* level in viewing the world. Knowing the landscape, faculty crafted the courses to help students develop an ethic of practice that was hardly enough to stand the pressures of the work environment ahead. The book, *Can Ethics Be Taught?*, tells the 5-year story of how this was achieved.

Such a conversation has not taken place in nursing, and certainly not in undergraduate nursing. However, we hope it will happen with the ideas presented in this text. Although it is true that nursing education has laudably embraced best practices and a strong commitment to teaching excellence within the last decade (Adams & Valiga, 2009; Shultz, 2009), this is not the entire reality. Because of the speed of change around us, many of the rules have changed and, as Parks (2000) said, students will follow the conventional ethos if it works for them. Developing and maintaining one's own personal professional ideal is not sufficient for professional education or membership, and steps must be taken by faculty to responsibly communicate this sea change to help move students to a level of critical–systemic thinking.

Trend #6: Taking Our Place at the Table: The Carnegie Study of Nursing Education

A singular theme emerged from the Carnegie Foundation for the Advancement of Teaching Study of Nursing Education (Benner et al., 2010) that did not appear in any of the other four *Preparation for the Professions* reports: Nursing education, pedagogically and curricularly, needs to take its place at the table. In five of the six recommendations, nursing is called to be a more active member of the academy and deliberately engage in multidisciplinary discussions about pedagogy, curriculum structure, and new research on how people learn.

The sixth recommendation continued with a "live larger" theme: move beyond the notion of socialization and the social paradigm of role taking, and *begin to actively think through and apply the notion of formation* (Benner et al., 2010, p. 390). Nursing education will need to think past the basics of critical thinking as a chic word to use and become facile with multiple ways of thinking; dialogical discourse needs to replace traditional didactic approaches; and, in the area of formation, nursing education is to move beyond the social constructs of *socialization and role taking* to *formation*. Without question, working with students in a profession to develop professional role identity is a formidable task. It will take intentional curriculum work, faculty development, and a commitment to new ways of thinking about professional role. The Carnegie Foundation's study of engineering affirmed that educators should envision students as young professionals, not just as students in the classroom; however, the message to engineering faculty was not the same as that for nursing. Benner et al. (2010) strongly argued that in order for our discipline to sit at the same table as professionals from law, ministry, engineering, and medicine, nursing and nursing education needs to be resculpted with a much larger, more sophisticated approach.

FOCUS ON THE NURSE PROFESSIONAL AS FITTING

These trends represent a vision of the future within the discipline that specifically address the demand for continuous relevance of the internal (nursing) environment. In the next section the authors discuss what a larger, more sophisticated approach would look like from the perspective of the external environment—specifically, the academy, the professions, and society.

Fit Within the Academy

Benner et al.'s (2010) work with the Carnegie Foundation and the inclusion of nursing as one of the five professions studied is a tremendous advantage to the discipline of nursing. Able thinkers and researchers like Benner offer legitimacy to nursing and to the research process, putting the discipline of nursing on the national stage. For the moment, the discipline's acceptance by the academic community as a full-fledged academic discipline is high. Unfortunately, professional ethics, like many other fields, had for years been preoccupied with decision-making bioethics and moral reasoning. Though other academic disciplines began to explore virtue ethics and professional education in the last several decades, American nursing interest in the topic has been minimal.

Most American ethics literature of the last 10 years focused on explication of the American Nurses Association's (ANA) code for nurses and other smaller works, whereas global interest in virtue ethics and professionalism in nursing greatly expanded. Sylvester (2002) argues that a top tier, or "learned-service" profession, must have an adequate level of ethical development so that the practitioners are "sufficiently [morally] mature to meet the demands of such a calling" (p. 314).

The Carnegie Foundation's emphasis on formation now makes clear to the nursing community that it is time to widen the conversation on exactly how professional formation can be described, defined, and assessed. Alignment within the academy means a continued commitment to ethical development and discourse surrounding the formation of professional identity. Two recent texts on excellence in nursing education (Adams & Valiga, 2009; Schultz, 2009) do not include ethics in either index. Viewing excellence only through pedagogical, business, or research lenses could be dangerous for the development of the profession.

Fit Within the Professions

Nursing is a moral endeavor (Bishop & Scudder, 1996; Vanlaere & Gastmans, 2007) in that the products of the profession serve the public good. People feel they can consistently trust nurses to act ethically (ANA, 2009) because being part of a profession "demands an uncommon insight and competence" (Sylvester, 2002, p. 315). Because professions incorporate practice, MacIntyre's (1984) characterization of a practice community as one that determines not only the appropriate technical standards but also, and more significantly, its normative standards, including the moral ends and means of practice. Alignment with such standards, ends, and means is extremely important.

The idea of professions as a *calling* is a substantive component of the Carnegie studies of law, medicine, ministry, and engineering, but is largely absent from nursing literature, and even from the Carnegie study of nursing education report (Benner, et al., 2010). For Sylvester (2002), the term *calling* equals the term *moral life*; this *moral life* cannot take root and flourish without a steady supply of ethical discourse. Perhaps the term has fallen out of favor because of a more competency, skills, and standards orientation for nursing in the last two decades. If this is the case, then it becomes even more problematic because a learned-service profession that is reduced to tasks and skills runs the risk of not continuing as part of first tier of professions. In the early 2000s colleagues in medicine adopted an outcome-based, assessment approach to professionalism without a coherent, mutually agreed upon curriculum, and found themselves with a plethora of instruments and few faculty development resources (Kao, Lim, Spevick, & Barzansky, 2003).

Perhaps nursing can learn from medicine and adopt more of a common approach that foundationally grounds students and faculty in a balanced, unified framework—the result the authors hope for with this work. Perhaps it is time to recast the language into a cohesive frame for thinking, proposed by the FrNP and the Stairstep model. These radical shifts from a fragmented conception of professionalism to a cohesive integrated whole represent a dramatic change. Using the term "calling" does not automatically lead one to a religious place for the other professions, and therefore should be fully appropriate to use when referring to nursing. Though others the discipline of nursing see the term as central to an accurate explanation of professionalism (Parks, 1993, 2000;

Sylvester, 2002), this work sees calling necessarily as part of a large conceptualization of professionalism, and unable to stand alone.

Fit Within Society

Since nurses are the most trusted professionals (ANA, 2009) and our visibility as a profession is better than it has ever been; discipline leaders need to carefully connect the idea of alignment or fit with society as a whole. The need for additional nurse practitioners as health care is extended to more Americans is a perfect opportunity to clarify the message about nursing as a respected, valued profession. Attention to the notion of fit or alignment will help those involved in crafting nursing's words to move away from identity descriptors and focus clearly on explaining nursing's impact and the ways that nursing can make a difference in people's lives. The fittingness extends globally to the migrant subcultures and care of diverse groups that are nested within a culture to situations in which nurses mobilize to other cultures and they themselves become members of a subculture. There is the ever present tension between multiculturalism and universal response (Crigger, Holcomb, & Weiss, 2001).

A collectively adopted and more explicit characterization of professionalism as a way of living life within a profession accommodates fledgling nurse professionals as well as those with many years of experience. Conceptual clarity (Porter-O'Grady & Malloch, 2009) will be increasingly important as the formation of nurse professionals becomes a more vital part of the discipline of nursing.

NEXT STEPS FOR NURSING EDUCATION

It is the authors' conclusion that nursing faculty and students seek a clearer and deeper understanding of formation for nurse professionals and that a singular focus on skills and competencies minimizes the goals and aspirations of those who choose nursing as their profession. These steps would substantially move the discipline forward in terms of professional formation.

1. *Adopt a framework for what professionalism is and how to become a nurse professional.* Using the FrNP to more completely conceptualize how one becomes a nurse professional and the Stairstep model to communicate how transformation takes place throughout one's professional life provides a fluid, redemptive way to look at professionalism in nursing. The authors have come to believe that this work is an important beginning in which new language and a stronger philosophical foundation can be helpful in nursing's further development as a discipline and a profession. Any framework or model should be practical. We believe that both the FrNP and the Stairstep model are simple and easy to communicate—and, most importantly, would give voice to how a nurse dialogically functions in practice using *phronesis*, or practical wisdom, to flourish.

Finally, the notion of flourishing adds a positive, hopeful dimension to what can often be a demanding profession.

2. *Anchor virtue ethics terms within a theoretical context specific to nursing.* Benner et al. (2010) found that students in the exemplar schools in the Carnegie study of nursing education used terms like *the good* in describing their nursing work. *Calling, virtue, ideal,* and *moral life* are other words that can reenter the nurse professional's vocabulary when connected with a larger view of what it means to be a nurse professional.

3. *Encourage the discourse needed to move the discipline forward.* The use of literature and writing to stimulate critical inquiry is important in developing a critical–systemic viewpoint. As Parks (1993) noted, a reflective–personal view—as opposed to a critical–systemic perspective—cannot adequately prepare students in the professions for the demands of their chosen field. A broader focus on what it means to help students move to a critical–systemic view needs to be part of disciplinary discourse, and, in turn, extended to how the profession is explicitly communicated to students within curricula. Explicit plans for facilitating learning are needed to engage students and move them beyond their conventional ethos.

4. *Integrate nursing education with liberal arts and multidisciplinary sources of influence.* No discipline can be rich if its members are marooned in a stagnated or underdeveloped point of view. The academic discipline and profession of nursing can only benefit from a wider view. Colleagues in arts and sciences and in other disciplines can broaden our own understanding of the nursing profession; as teachers, contact with other academic colleagues should not be limited to sharing teaching strategies.

CHALLENGES FOR THE FUTURE

As we look to the future of nursing and of nurse professionals, there are two additional concerns about professional education that are worthy of note. Distance learning and online courses have revolutionized academic education. Surprisingly, little research has been conducted to determine the impact of distance learning on professional development, and the concern is that e-learning may not be as effective as other methods in developing nurse professionals (Faison, 2003). Rieck and Crouch (2007) suggest that online learning may challenge learners' abilities to connect socially and may increase incivility. If professional development occurs mainly in the clinical settings as suggested (Benner et al., 2010), how significant is face-to-face contact in professional development and professional education?

Globalization will continue to impact nursing education. Migrated students and nurses challenge educators to properly balance students' cultural beliefs and values while educating them to become nurse professionals. International travel, service learning, and a growing desire for a cosmopolitan education that encourages the proper use of humility will become more prominent in the educational landscape.

CONCLUSION

How do nurse educators contribute to the making of nurse professionals? We believe that nurse educators can bring together the rich heritage of professionalism and recent work within a variety of disciplines to develop more effective curricula for educating nurse professionals. The making of nurse professionals is a transformational process that begins with the education of a good nurse who practices the profession well throughout a lifetime. We believe that one way to accomplish this task begins with a reframing of professionalism and professional ethics. By conceiving the profession and *what it means to be a nurse professional* in a more robust and balanced, psychological/social view, nurses can truly flourish as lifelong contributors in a vibrant and rewarding profession.

REFERENCES

Adams, M. H., & Valiga, T. M. (2009). *Achieving excellence in nursing education*. New York: National League for Nursing.

American Nurses Association. (2009). *Gallup poll votes nurses most trusted profession*. Available online at http://www.medicalnewstoday.com/articles/173627.php. Retrieved January 23, 2010.

Benner, P., Sutphen, M., Leonard-Kahn, V., & Day, L. (2010). *Educating nurses: A call for radical transformation*. San Francisco: Jossey-Bass and Stanford, CA: The Carnegie Foundation for the Advancement of Teaching and Learning.

Bishop, A. H., & Scudder, J. R. (1996). *Nursing ethics: Therapeutic caring presence*. Sudbury, MA: Jones and Bartlett.

Covey, S. R. (1994). *First things first*. New York: Covey Leadership Center.

Crigger, N. J., Holcomb, L., & Weiss, J. (2001). Fundamentalism, multiculturalism and problems of conducting research with populations in developing nations. *Nursing Ethics*, *8*(5), 459–468.

Faison, K. A. (2003). Professionalization in a distance learning setting. *The Association of Black Nursing Faculty Journal*, July/August, 83–85.

Giddens, J. F., & Brady, D. P. (2007). Rescuing nursing education from content saturation: The case for a concept-based curriculum. *Journal of Nursing Education*, *46*(2), 65–69.

Kao, A., Lim, M., Spevick, J., & Barzansky, B. (2003). Teaching and evaluating students' professionalism in US medical schools, 2002–2003. *Journal of the American Medical Association*, *290*(9), 1151–1152.

Lave, J., & Wenger, E. (1991). *Situated learning: Legitimate peripheral participation*. New York: Cambridge University Press.

MacIntyre, A. (1984). *After virtue* (2nd ed.). Notre Dame, IN: University of Notre Dame Press.

Parks, S. D. (1993). Is it too late? Young adults and the formation of professional ethics. In T. R. Piper, M. C. Gentile, & S. D. Parks (Eds.), *Can ethics be taught? Perspectives, challenges, and approaches at Harvard Business School* (pp. 13–72). Boston: Harvard Business School.

Parks, S. D. (2000). *Big questions, worthy dreams: Mentoring young adults in their search for meaning, purpose and faith.* San Francisco: Jossey-Bass.

Porter-O'Grady, T. (2009). *Healthcare 2010 and beyond.* Lessons from Legends Series, University of Kansas School of Nursing, November 6, 2010.

Porter-O'Grady, T., & Malloch, K. (2009). Leaders of innovation: Transforming postindustrial healthcare. *Journal of Nursing Administration, 39*(6), 245–248.

Rieck, S., & Crouch, L. (2007). Connectiveness and civility in online learning. *Nurse Education in Practice, 7*, 425–432.

Ross, A. M., Noone, J., Luce, L., & Sideras, S. (2009). Spiraling evidence-based practice and outcomes management concepts in an undergraduate curriculum: A systematic approach. *Journal of Nursing Education, 48*(6), 319–326.

Shultz, C. M. (2009). *Building a science of nursing education: Foundation for evidence-based teaching-learning.* New York: National League for Nursing.

Sylvester, C. (2002). Ethics and the quest for professionalization. *Therapeutic Recreation Journal, 36*(4), 314–334.

Vacek, J. E. (2009). Using a conceptual approach with concept mapping to promote critical thinking. *Journal of Nursing Education, 48*(1), 45–48.

Vanlaere, L., & Gastmans, C. (2007). Ethics in nursing education: Learning to reflect on care practices. *Nursing Ethics, 14*(6), 758–766.

Index

Note: Page numbers followed by *f* indicate figures and those followed by *t* indicate tables.

141